World Health Organization

The series *International Histological Classification of Tumours* consists of the following volumes. Each of these volumes - apart from volumes 1 and 2, which have already been revised - will appear in a revised edition within the next few years. Volumes of the current editions can be ordered through WHO, Distribution and Sales, Avenue Appia, CH-1211 Geneva 27.

1. Histological typing of lung tumours (1967, second edition 1981)
2. Histological typing of breast tumours (1968, second edition 1981)
3. Histological typing of soft tissue tumours (1969)
4. Histological typing of oral and oropharyngeal tumours (1971)
5. Histological typing of odontogenic tumours, jaw cysts, and allied lesions (1971)
6. Histological typing of bone tumours (1972)
7. Histological typing of salivary gland tumours (1972)
8. Cytology of the female genital tract (1973)
9. Histological typing of ovarian tumours (1973)
10. Histological typing of urinary bladder tumours (1973)
12. Histological typing of skin tumours (1974)
13. Histological typing of female genital tract tumours (1975)
14. Histological and cytological typing of neoplastic diseases of haematopoietic and lymphoid tissues (1976)
16. Histological typing of testis tumours (1977)
17. Cytology of non-gynaecological sites (1977)
19. Histological typing of upper respiratory tract tumours (1978)
20. Histological typing of tumours of the liver, biliary tract and pancreas (1978)
21. Histological typing of tumours of the central nervous system (1979)
22. Histological typing of prostate tumours (1980)
23. Histological typing of endocrine tumours (1980)
24. Histological typing of tumours of the eye and its adnexa (1980)
25. Histological typing of kidney tumours (1981)

A coded compendium of the International Histological Classification of Tumours (1978).

The following volumes have already appeared in a revised edition with Springer-Verlag:

Histological Typing of Thyroid Tumours, 2nd edn. Hedinger/Williams/Sobin (1988)

Histological Typing of Intestinal Tumours, 2nd edn. Jass/Sobin (1989)

Histological Typing of Oesophageal and Gastric Tumours, 2nd edn. Watanabe/Jass/Sobin (1990)

In this series, colour illustrations will be limited in number in order to maintain a reasonable sales price.

A set of 120 colour slides (35 mm), corresponding to the photomicrographs in the book, is available from the American Registry of Pathology, 14th Street and Alaska Ave. NW, Washington, DC 20306, USA. For further information please see p. 109.

Histological Typing of Oesophageal and Gastric Tumours

H. Watanabe, J. R. Jass, and L. H. Sobin

In Collaboration with
Pathologists in 8 Countries

Second Edition

With 120 Figures

Springer-Verlag Berlin Heidelberg New York
London Paris Tokyo Hong Kong

H. Watanabe
1st Department of Pathology, Niigata University School of Medicine
Niigata, Japan

J. R. Jass
WHO Collaborating Centre
for the Histological Classification of Intestinal Tumours
Department of Pathology, St. Mark's Hospital, London, UK
and present address:
Department of Pathology, University of Auckland, School of Medicine
Auckland, New Zealand

L. H. Sobin
Department of Gastrointestinal Pathology and WHO Collaborating Centre
for the International Histological Classification of Tumours, Armed Forces
Institute of Pathology, Washington, DC, USA

First edition published by WHO in 1977 as No. 18 in the International Histological Classification of Tumours series

ISBN-13:978-3-540-51629-3 **e-ISBN-13:978-3-642-83920-7**
DOI: 10.1007/978-3-642-83920-7

Library of Congress Cataloging-in-Publication Data. Watanabe, H. (Hidenobu)
Histological typing of oesophageal and gastric tumours/H. Watanabe, J. R. Jass, and L. H Sobin, in collaboration with pathologists in 8 countries. – 2nd ed. p. cm – (International histological classification of tumours) Rev. ed. of: Histological typing of gastric and oesophageal tumours/K. Oota, in collaboration with L. H. Sobin and pathologists in thirteen countries. 1977
ISBN 0-387-51629-8 (U.S.)
1. Stomach–Tumors–Histopathology–Classification. 2. Esophagus–Tumors–Histopathology–Classification. I. Jass, Jeremy R. II. Sobin, L. H III. Oota, Kunio, 1913– Histological typing of gastric and oesophageal tumours. IV. Title V. Series.
[DNLM: 1. Esophageal Neoplasms–classification. 2. Esophageal Neoplasms–pathology. 3. Stomach Neoplasms–classification. 4 Stomach Neoplasms–pathology. W1 IN764G/W1 15 W324h] RC258.I45 no. 18. 1990 [RC280.S8] 616.99'207583 s–dc20 [616.99'233] DNLM/DLC for Library of Congress 90-9472 CIP

Softcover reprint of the hardcover 2nd edition 1990

Typesetting, printing and binding: Appl, Wemding
2121/3145-543210 – Printed on acid-free paper

General Preface to the Series

Among the prerequisites for comparative studies of cancer are international agreement on histological criteria for the definition and classification of cancer types and a standardized nomenclature. An internationally agreed classification of tumours, acceptable alike to physicians, surgeons, radiologists, pathologists and statisticians, would enable cancer workers in all parts of the world to compare their findings and would facilitate collaboration among them.

In a report published in 1952,[1] a subcommittee of the World Health Organization (WHO) Expert Committee on Health Statistics discussed the general principles that should govern the statistical classification of tumours and agreed that, to ensure the necessary flexibility and ease of coding, three separate classifications were needed according to (1) anatomical site, (2) histological type, and (3) degree of malignancy. A classification according to anatomical site is available in the International Classification of Diseases.[2]

In 1956, the WHO Executive Board passed a resolution[3] requesting the Director-General to explore the possibility that WHO might organize centres in various parts of the world and arrange for the collection of human tissues and their histological classification. The main purpose of such centres would be to develop histological definitions of cancer types and to facilitate the wide adoption of a uniform nomenclature. The resolution was endorsed by the Tenth World Health Assembly in May 1957.[4]

---

[1] WHO (1952) WHO Technical Report Series. No. 53, 1952, p 45

[2] WHO (1977) Manual of the international statistical classification of diseases, injuries, and causes of death. 1975 version Geneva

[3] WHO (1956) WHO Official Records. No. 68, p 14 (resolution EB 17.R40)

[4] WHO (1957) WHO Official Records. No. 79, p 467 (resolution WHA 10.18)

Since 1958, WHO has established a number of centres concerned with this subject. The result of this endeavour has been the International Histological Classification of Tumours, a multivolumed series whose first edition was published between 1967 and 1981. The present revised second edition aims to update the classification, reflecting progress in diagnosis and the relevance of tumour types to clinical and epidemiological features.

Preface to Histological Typing of Oesophageal and Gastric Tumours, Second Edition

The first edition of *Histological Typing of Gastric and Oesophageal Tumours*[1] was the result of a collaborative effort organized by WHO and carried out by the International Reference/Collaborating Centre for the Histological Classification of Gastric and Oesophageal Tumours at the Department of Pathology, Faculty of Medicine, University of Tokyo, Japan.

In order to keep the classification up to date, a set of revision proposals was circulated to the participants listed on pages XI and XII. Their responses provided the basis for a new draft. After further communications among the participants, the present classification, definitions and explanatory notes were recommended for publication.

The histological classification of oesophageal and gastric tumours, which appears on pages 5–9, contains the morphology code numbers of the International Classification of Diseases for Oncology (ICD-O)[2] and the Systematized Nomenclature of Medicine (SNOMED).[3]

It will, of course, be appreciated that the classification reflects the present state of knowledge, and modifications are almost certain to be needed as experience accumulates. Although the present classification has been adopted by the members of the group, it necessarily represents a view from which some pathologists may wish to dissent.

---

1 Oota K, Sobin LH (1977) Histological Typing of Gastric and Oesophageal Tumours. Geneva, World Health Organization (International Histological Classification of Tumours, No. 18)

2 World Health Organization (1976) International Classification of Diseases for Oncology. Geneva

3 College of American Pathologists (1976) Systematized Nomenclature of Medicine. Chicago

It is nevertheless hoped that, in the interests of international cooperation, all pathologists will use the classification as put forward. Criticism and suggestions for its improvement will be welcomed; these should be sent to the World Health Organization, Geneva, Switzerland.

The publications in the series *International Histological Classification of Tumours* are not intended to serve as textbooks but rather to promote the adoption of a uniform terminology that will facilitate communication among cancer workers. For this reason the literature references have intentionally been omitted and readers should refer to standard works for bibliographies.

Table of Contents

Participants

Cuvelier, C., Dr.
Department of Pathology, University Hospital, Ghent, Belgium

Fenger, C., Dr.
Universitetets Patologiske Institut, Odense Sygehus, Odense, Denmark

Hermanek, P., Dr.
Abteilung für Klinische Pathologie, Chirurgische Klinik mit Poliklinik der Universität Erlangen-Nürnberg, Erlangen, Federal Republic of Germany

Jass, J.R., Dr.
Department of Pathology, St. Mark's Hospital, London, United Kingdom. (WHO Collaborating Centre for the Histological Classification of Intestinal Tumours). Present address: Department of Pathology, University of Auckland School of Medicine, Auckland, New Zealand

Ming, S.-C., Dr.
Department of Pathology, Temple University School of Medicine, Philadelphia, Pa, USA

Newland, R.C., Dr.
Anatomical Pathology, Repatriation General Hospital Concord, Concord, NSW, Australia

Sipponen, P., Dr.
Department of Pathology, Jorvi Hospital, Espoo, Finland

Sobin, L. H., Dr.
Department of Gastrointestinal Pathology, Armed Forces Institute of Pathology, Washington, DC, USA. (WHO Collaborating Centre for the International Histological Classification of Tumours)

Wang, R.-N., Dr.
Department of Pathologic Anatomy, Shanghai Second Medical University, Shanghai, China

Watanabe, H., Dr.
1st Department of Pathology, Niigata University School of Medicine, Niigata, Japan

Williams, E. D., Dr.
Department of Pathology, University Hospital of Wales, Cardiff, Wales. (WHO Collaborating Centre for the Histological Classification of Endocrine Tumours)

Introduction

This classification is based primarily on the microscopic characteristics of tumours. It is therefore concerned with the identification of cell types and histological patterns as seen by conventional light microscopy. In general, time-honoured terms have been retained. Synonyms are listed only if they have been widely used, or if they are considered to be important for understanding the disease process. In such cases the preferred term is given first, followed by the synonym in parentheses.

The individuality of the tumour manifests itself principally in its histological appearance and the extent of spread at the time of diagnosis. This volume is concerned only with the histological classification of tumours. Anatomical extent or staging is covered in the *TNM Classification.*[1]

The histological classification of a tumour depends on two main parameters, typing and grading, and a number of additional parameters which may apply to selected examples.

Histological Typing

Histological typing divides tumours of a given organ into different types according to their direction of differentiation. Although this may frequently indicate the underlying histogenesis of the tumour, it may in some cases be difficult or impossible to be certain as to the cell of origin. Note is taken of the structure and function of cell types as well as the overall growth pattern of the tumour, with the aim of

---

[1] International Union Against Cancer (1987) TNM Classification of Malignant Tumours, 4th edn. Hermanek P, Sobin LH (eds). Springer, Berlin Heidelberg New York

matching these features to those of a normal tissue found in the same organ.

Malignant tumours, especially carcinomas of the stomach, may contain areas of different histological types. Such tumours should be first categorized according to the predominant histological type and notes added indicating the presence of other histological types.

Histological Grading

Grading of tumours of the same histological type is performed to provide some indication of their aggressiveness, which may in turn relate to prognosis or treatment. Here one considers the degree of cytological and architectural similarity to the presumed tissue of origin, as well as nuclear abnormalities and mitotic activity. Four categories may be distinguished:

Well differentiated: a carcinoma with histological and cellular features that closely resemble those of normal epithelium of similar type
Moderately differentiated: a carcinoma intermediate between well differentiated and poorly differentiated.
Poorly differentiated: a carcinoma with histological and cellular features that only barely resemble those of normal epithelium of similar type.
Undifferentiated: a carcinoma with no glandular or squamous structure or other features to indicate definite differentiation.

Well and moderately differentiated tumours can be grouped together as low grade, and poorly differentiated and undifferentiated as high grade. When a tumour shows different grades of differentiation, the higher grade should determine the final categorization. Grading and typing should not be made, however, at the advancing margins of the tumour or at the portions directly adjacent to ulcerative or inflammatory processes.

Additional Histological Parameters

In certain types of tumour additional histological parameters may be important. These include the deepest anatomical layer of the wall invaded by the tumour, the character of invasive margin (expanding or well-circumscribed versus diffusely infiltrating), inflammatory cell reaction, fibrous (desmoplastic) reaction, invasion of lymphatics, vessels or perineural spaces, and the type of lymph node reaction. Some of these features may assume clinical importance, particularly if they are shown to have a significant and independent influence upon prognosis.

Precancerous Lesions and Dysplasia

Screening and follow-up surveillance of high-risk groups of patients can play an important role in the prevention and control of cancer. The recognition of a histopathological abnormality that is more likely to develop into cancer than its normal counterpart represents a key factor in the prevention of cancer. Such an abnormality is known as a precancerous lesion. This should be distinguished from a precancerous condition, which is a clinical state associated with an increased risk of cancer. The term 'precancerous' does not imply that malignant progression is inevitable; rather, it is a marker of an increased probability of malignant change. It also does not imply that all cancers must necessarily develop within a precancerous lesion.

The term 'dysplasia' can be used to describe most precancerous epithelial lesions. Some prefer to use the term 'atypia', although this term has usually been restricted to the description of cytological abnormalities. Dysplasia encompasses changes in architecture and aberrant differentiation as well as cytological disturbances and therefore has a broad meaning. The classical and most usual manifestation of gastrointestinal dysplasia is as a circumscribed lesion, i. e. an adenoma. Particular problems concern distinguishing between dysplasia and reactive, regenerative or degenerative changes, and also between dysplasia and carcinoma in situ or intramucosal carcinoma, and the grading of dysplasia. Making these distinctions may be difficult in some cases, especially on the basis of endoscopic biopsy.

It should be stressed that the term 'dysplasia' should only be applied to the description of cytological and architectural changes in lesions that are considered to be precancerous and is only appropriate when there is no evidence of invasion. The diagnosis does not exclude the possibility of a co-existing carcinoma, which emphasizes the importance of placing histopathological reporting into the clinical context, particularly because of the difficulty of reaching a definitive decision on the benign or malignant nature of some lesions on the basis of endoscopic biopsy.

Histological Classification of Oesophageal Tumours

1	**Epithelial tumours**	
1.1	*Benign*	
1.1.1	Squamous cell papilloma	8052/0[a]
1.1.2	Viral wart	76600
1.1.3	Adenoma	8140/0
1.2	*Malignant*	
1.2.1	Squamous cell carcinoma	8070/3
1.2.2	Verrucous (squamous) carcinoma	8051/3
1.2.3	Spindle cell (squamous) carcinoma	8074/3
1.2.4	Adenocarcinoma	8140/3
1.2.5	Adenosquamous carcinoma	8560/3
1.2.6	Mucoepidermoid carcinoma	8430/3
1.2.7	Adenoid cystic carcinoma	8200/3
1.2.8	Small cell carcinoma	8041/3
1.2.9	Undifferentiated carcinoma	8020/3
1.2.10	Others	
2	**Non-epithelial tumours**	
2.1	*Benign*	
2.1.1	Leiomyoma	8890/0
2.1.2	Lipoma	8850/0
2.1.3	Vascular tumours	

[a] Morphology code of the International Classification of Diseases for Oncology (ICD-O) and the Systematized Nomenclature of Medicine (SNOMED)

2.1.4	Neurogenic tumours	
2.1.4.1	Granular cell tumour	9580/0
2.1.4.2	Others	
2.1.5	Others	
2.2	*Malignant*	
2.2.1	Leiomyosarcoma	8890/3
2.2.2	Kaposi sarcoma	9140/3
2.2.3	Others	
3	**Miscellaneous tumours**	
3.1	*Carcinosarcoma*	8980/3
3.2	*Malignant melanoma*	8720/3
3.3	*Others*	
3.3.1	Carcinoid tumour	8240/3
3.3.2	Malignant lymphoma	9590/3
4	**Secondary tumours**	
5	**Tumour-like lesions**	
5.1	*Fibrovascular (fibrous) polyp*	76806
5.2	*Cysts*	33400
5.2.1	Congenital cysts	26500
5.2.2	Retention cyst	33730
5.3	*Inflammatory polyp*	76820
5.4	*Glycogenic acanthosis*	
5.5	*Diffuse leiomyomatosis*	
5.6	*Gastric heterotopia*	26080
6	**Epithelial abnormalities (precancerous)**	
6.1	*Dysplasia and carcinoma in situ in squamous epithelium*	74000
6.2	*Barrett oesophagus*	73330
6.3	*Dysplasia in columnar epithelium (Barrett oesophagus)*	74000

Histological Classification of Gastric Tumours

1	**Epithelial tumours**	
1.1	*Benign*	
1.1.1	Adenoma	8140/0
1.1.1.1	Tubular adenoma	8211/0
1.1.1.2	Villous adenoma	8261/0
1.1.1.3	Tubulovillous adenoma	8263/0
1.2	*Malignant*	
1.2.1	Adenocarcinoma	8140/3
1.2.1.1	Papillary adenocarcinoma	8260/3
1.2.1.2	Tubular adenocarcinoma	8211/3
1.2.1.3	Mucinous adenocarcinoma	8480/3
1.2.1.4	Signet-ring cell carcinoma	8490/3
1.2.2	Adenosquamous carcinoma	8560/3
1.2.3	Squamous cell carcinoma	8070/3
1.2.4	Small cell carcinoma	8041/3
1.2.5	Undifferentiated carcinoma	8020/3
1.2.6	Others	
2	**Endocrine tumours**	
2.1	*Carcinoid tumour*	8240/3
2.2	*Mixed carcinoid-adenocarcinoma*	8244/3
3	**Non-epithelial tumours**	
3.1	*Benign*	
3.1.1	Leiomyoma	8890/0
3.1.2	Lipoma	8850/0

3.1.3	Vascular tumours	
3.1.3.1	Haemangioma	9120/0
3.1.3.2	Lymphangioma	9170/0
3.1.3.3	Glomus tumour	8711/0
3.1.4	Neurogenic tumours	
3.1.4.1	Neurilemmoma (schwannoma)	9560/0
3.1.4.2	Neurofibroma	9540/0
3.1.4.3	Granular cell tumour	9580/0
3.1.5	Others	
3.2	*Malignant*	
3.2.1	Leiomyosarcoma	8890/3
3.2.2	Kaposi sarcoma	9140/3
3.2.3	Malignant neurilemmoma (malignant schwannoma, neurogenic sarcoma)	9560/3
3.2.4	Others	
4	**Malignant lymphomas**	
5	**Miscellaneous tumours**	
6	**Secondary tumours**	
7	**Tumour-like lesions**	
7.1	*Hyperplastic polyp*	72040
7.2	*Hamartomas*	75500
7.2.1	Fundic gland polyp and polyposis	
7.2.2	Peutz-Jeghers polyp and polyposis	75630
7.2.3	Juvenile polyp and polyposis	75640
7.3	*Heterotopias*	
7.3.1	Pancreatic heterotopia	26020
7.3.2	Gastric gland heterotopia	26080
7.4	*Hypertrophic rugal lesions*	
7.4.1	Giant rugal hypertrophy (Ménétrier disease)	71330
7.4.2	Fundic gland hyperplasia (Zollinger-Ellison syndrome)	72420
7.4.3	Gastritis cystica polyposa (stomal polypoid hypertrophic gastritis)	72040

7.5	*Cronkhite-Canada polyposis*	
7.6	*Inflammatory fibroid polyp*	76830
7.7	*Endocrine cell hyperplasia and micronest*	
7.8	*Benign lymphoid hyperplasia*	72200
7.9	*Others*	

8 **Epithelial abnormalities (precancerous)**

8.1	*Dysplasia*	74000

Definitions and Explanatory Notes

Oesophagus

1 Epithelial Tumours

1.1 Benign

1.1.1 Squamous Cell Papilloma (Figs. 1, 2)

A benign tumour composed of hyperplastic squamous epithelium covering finger-like processes with cores derived from the lamina propria.

This is rare. There is an extremely rare inherited condition of multiple papillomas of the oesophagus in association with hyperkeratosis of the palms and soles. Multiple papillomas of the oesophagus have also been found in patients with acanthosis nigricans.

1.1.2 Viral Wart

A squamous cell papilloma associated with human papilloma virus.

These lesions are multiple and akin to those seen in the upper respiratory tract. They are rare.

1.1.3 Adenoma

Adenomas are essentially restricted to Barrett oesophagus where they are usually polypoid. They are rare.

1.2 Malignant

1.2.1 Squamous Cell Carcinoma (Figs. 3–7)

A malignant tumour composed of squamous-type epithelium.

This is the most common malignant tumour of the oesophagus. It is usually graded as well, moderately or poorly differentiated. Well differentiated tumours are those with abundant amounts of keratin, easily demonstrated intercellular bridges and cell layers undergoing differentiation. Poorly differentiated tumours are those with little or no keratin, intercellular bridges and differentiation of cell layers. Moderately differentiated tumours are those intermediate between well and poorly differentiated.

After radiotherapy or chemotherapy squamous cell carcinomas usually show characteristic changes in their histological appearances. Loss or loosening of cell cohesion with degenerative atypia may be seen as an early response. Later, the tumour cells may disappear almost completely, leaving fibrotic areas in which small groups of bizarre eosinophilic cells containing pyknotic or fragmented nuclei are embedded. There may be a foreign body granulomatous response around keratinized material. Recurrent tumour cells may appear undifferentiated.

1.2.2 Verrucous (Squamous) Carcinoma (Figs. 8, 9)

A malignant papillary tumour composed of well-differentiated squamous epithelium with minimal cytological atypia and blunt, pushing margins rather than insinuating, tentacular growth.

This is a rare variant of well-differentiated squamous cell carcinoma.

1.2.3 Spindle Cell (Squamous) Carcinoma (Figs. 10–13)

A squamous cell carcinoma consisting largely or wholly of spindle-shaped cells.

A variant of poorly differentiated squamous cell carcinoma, this tumour may be mistaken for a sarcoma or carcinosarcoma. However, special techniques such as electron microscopy and immunohistochemistry may reveal the spindle cells to be variants of squamous cells. They are usually polypoid and contain areas of squamous cell carcinoma in situ or nests of squamous cells in various degrees of differentiation embedded in a stroma composed of atypical fibroblasts. This has been described as a pseudosarcoma or pseudosarcomatous carcinoma in the past (Figs. 12, 13). The proportions of epithelial and stromal components can vary in different cases.

1.2.4 Adenocarcinoma (Figs. 14, 15)

A malignant tumour composed of glandular epithelium, with papillary and/or tubular structures.

Most oesophageal adenocarcinomas arise in metaplastic glandular mucosa of Barrett oesophagus, a sequel to prolonged reflux oesophagitis. They occur in the lower portion of the oesophagus and may or may not be preceded by dysplasia (Sects. 6.2, 6.3). Primary adenocarcinoma can arise from congenital heterotopic gastric mucosa. Such foci are usually located in the upper oesophagus. Adenocarcinoma can also arise from oesophageal glands. It may be difficult or impossible to determine whether an advanced adenocarcinoma of the lower oesophagus is the result of spread from a tumour of the stomach or is a true primary growth of the oesophagus.

Adenocarcinomas with small foci of squamous metaplasia should be classified under adenocarcinoma with the squamous components referred to in the description.

1.2.5 Adenosquamous Carcinoma

A tumour in which adenocarcinomatous and squamous carcinomatous components are intermingled or have a fairly clear boundary.

The adenocarcinomatous component is usually tubular.

1.2.6 Mucoepidermoid Carcinoma (Figs. 16, 17)

A tumour characterized by the presence of an intimate mixture of squamous cells, mucus-secreting cells and cells of an intermediate type, the relative proportions of which vary.

The squamous cell component is usually present in the form of clumps or multilayered masses beneath the mucus-secreting epithelium. Keratinization is uncommon. These tumours are identical to the mucoepidermoid tumours of salivary glands but are usually of higher cytological grade. They are rare in the oesophagus and are believed to arise from oesophageal glands.

1.2.7 Adenoid Cystic Carcinoma (Figs. 18, 19)

A malignant epithelial tumour having a characteristic cribriform structure with tumour cells of two types - cells similar to those lining the normal mucous gland ducts and cells of myoepithelial type - which form small duct-like or trabecular structures or larger solid masses dispersed around cystic spaces, as in similar tumours of the salivary glands.

This tumour is rare in the oesophagus and is believed to arise from oesophageal glands. It sometimes has a high nuclear grade, especially in the large solid masses; such a tumor can simulate poorly differentiated squamous cell carcinoma, small cell carcinoma, or undifferentiated carcinoma.

1.2.8 Small Cell Carcinoma (Figs. 20-22)

A tumour that resembles the similarly named but very much more common tumour found in the lung in terms of its histology, immunohistochemistry, ultrastructure and clinical behaviour.

It is important to exclude secondary spread from a pulmonary source. Oesophageal small cell carcinomas may or may not contain signs of endocrine differentiation, e.g. dense core granules and argyrophilia. The carcinoma is pure in most cases, but may have foci of squamous cell carcinoma or rarely adenocarcinoma.

1.2.9 Undifferentiated Carcinoma

A malignant epithelial tumour that shows no glandular or squamous structure.

This should be distinguished from small cell carcinoma.

1.2.10 Others

Choriocarcinoma has been described in the oesophagus.

2 Non-epithelial Tumours

See *Histological Typing of Soft Tissues Tumours* for definitions and explanatory notes.

2.1 Benign

2.1.1 Leiomyoma

This is the most common type of benign non-epithelial tumour encountered in the oesophagus. It arises mostly from the muscle coat and less often from the muscularis mucosae.

2.1.2 Lipoma

2.1.3 Vascular Tumours

2.1.4 Neurogenic Tumours

2.1.4.1 Granular Cell Tumour
The oesophagus is a major site for the granular cell tumour in the digestive tract. It is usually located in the submucosa. Pseudoepitheliomatous hyperplasia of the overlying squamous epithelium may simulate carcinoma, especially on endoscopic biopsy. Granular cell tumours can be multiple.

2.1.4.2 Others
These include neurilemmoma (schwannoma) and neurofibroma.

2.1.5 Others

2.2 Malignant

2.2.1 Leiomyosarcoma

This is the most frequently encountered malignant non-epithelial tumour of the oesophagus. The distinction between benign and malignant smooth muscle tumours may not be straightforward. The most helpful pointers to malignancy are a high mitotic rate (more than 10 mitoses per 50 high-power fields), a high nucleocytoplasmic ratio, dense cellularity, large tumour size, invasion of adjacent structures and necrosis.

2.2.2 Kaposi sarcoma

This is largely associated with the acquired immune deficiency syndrome.

2.2.3 Others

3 Miscellaneous Tumours

3.1 Carcinosarcoma

A tumour comprising both carcinomatous and sarcomatous elements.

This is rare in the oesophagus. The carcinomatous part is usually squamous, and the sarcomatous components are heterologous (e.g. cartilage, bone, striated muscle). This tumour should be distinguished from spindle cell (squamous) carcinoma, namely by the specific differentiation in the sarcomatous component (Sect. 1.2.3).

3.2 Malignant Melanoma (Fig. 23)

Malignant melanoma in the oesophagus is much more commonly metastatic than primary. Junctional activity and an adjacent intra-epithelial component are important features of primary tumours, but they may be obscured in advanced disease.

3.3 Others

3.3.1 Carcinoid Tumour

These tumours rarely occur in the oesophagus. When they do, it is usually within the metaplastic glandular mucosa of Barrett oesophagus.

3.3.2 Malignant Lymphoma

4 Secondary Tumours

5 Tumour-like Lesions

5.1 Fibrovascular (Fibrous) Polyp

A polyp composed of a core of fibrous or fibro-adipose connective tissue and blood vessels covered by thickened but otherwise normal squamous epithelium.

This can achieve considerable length.

5.2 Cysts

5.2.1 Congenital Cysts

These malformations are lined either by epithelium that is columnar, ciliated columnar, squamous or gastric or by more than one of these. They can be subclassified into inclusion cyst and duplication cyst.

5.2.2 Retention Cyst

Cystic dilatation of the oesophageal glands as a result of obstruction or stenosis to glandular outflow, especially following stricture.

When a number of glands are involved, the lesion may simulate diverticula, so called pseudodiverticulosis.

5.3 Inflammatory Polyp

This is typically found in Barrett oesophagus.

5.4 Glycogenic Acanthosis (Fig. 24)

Multiple white plaques with squamous epithelium that is thickened and contains large glycogen-filled cells.

5.5 Diffuse Leiomyomatosis

A diffuse proliferation or hyperplasia of smooth muscle with a serpentine, whorled pattern rather than a solitary tumour mass.

The condition is probably a malformation or hamartoma. It typically presents in young adults. Leiomyomatosis may extend from the oesophagus to the stomach.

5.6 Gastric Heterotopia

Small islands of gastric heterotopia, usually fundic-type mucosa, in the upper oesophagus.

These may replace the oesophageal squamous epithelium or lie in the subepithelial tissue immediately beneath it.

6 Epithelial Abnormalities (Precancerous)

6.1 Dysplasia and Carcinoma In Situ in Squamous Epithelium (Figs. 25, 26)

Dysplasia of squamous epithelium of the oesophagus is similar to the more extensively investigated lesion encountered in the uterine cervix. Nuclei are enlarged and hyperchromatic and show increased mitotic activity. In mild dysplasia such atypical nuclei are limited to the basal zone, and there is evidence of cytoplasmic maturation superficially. With increasing grades of dysplasia there is a progressive increase in the proportion of atypical basal cells until the entire thickness of the mucosa is replaced. This state is described as carcinoma in situ.

Practical problems are the distinction between dysplasia, a precancerous lesion, and the much more frequently encountered inflammatory, regenerative and degenerative changes occurring in reflux or other forms of oesophagitis (Figs. 27-29). It may be particularly difficult to make this distinction in the presence of an actively inflamed or eroded lesion on endoscopic biopsy.

Leukoplakia, or white plaques, in the oesophagus may be associated with a variety of lesions including reflux oesophagitis, candidiasis, glycogenic acanthosis, lichen planus, dysplasia and carcinoma in situ. There is no evidence that precancerous leukoplakia as seen in the mouth, vulva or anal region occurs in the oesophagus.

6.2 Barrett Oesophagus (Fig. 30)

Glandular metaplasia of the oesophageal mucosa, typically a sequel to chronic reflux oesophagitis.

Two main types of glandular mucosa are seen in Barrett oesophagus: gastric and intestinal. The glandular mucosa may be flat or in elevated polypoid structures.

6.3 Dysplasia in Columnar Epithelium (Barrett Oesophagus)

This resembles dysplasia in the stomach ("Gastric Tumors", Sect. 8). It is graded as mild, moderate or severe, the first two comprising low-grade and the last, high-grade dysplasia. Distinction between the latter, adenocarcinoma in situ and intramucosal adenocarcinoma can be especially difficult on small, superficial endoscopic biopsies.

Dysplasia is the most reliable marker for assessing the risk of adenocarcinoma in the lower oesophagus. In fact, most adenocarcinomas of the oesophagus arise in patients with Barrett oesophagus. Dysplasia develops more frequently in the intestinal than in the gastric type of mucosa.

Stomach

1 Epithelial Tumours

1.1 Benign

1.1.1 Adenoma (Figs. 31–42)

A circumscribed benign neoplasm composed of tubular and/or villous structures lined by dysplastic epithelium.

1.1.1.1 Tubular Adenoma
An adenoma composed of tubules surrounded by lamina propria.

1.1.1.2 Villous Adenoma
An adenoma composed of blunt or pointed finger-like structures or folia with cores of lamina propria producing a papillary configuration.

1.1.1.3 Tubulovillous Adenoma
An adenoma composed of both tubular and villous structures, each contributing to more than 20% of the tumour.

This pattern has been known as papillotubular.

Although this classification is similar to that given in the volume on intestinal tumours, gastric adenomas differ in a number of respects from adenomas of the large intestine. Gastric tubular adenomas are more often slightly raised, sessile polypoid lesions than pedunculated.

They are sometimes flat, depressed, or volcano-like lesions (brown or yellow-brown when fixed) with a gyrus-like or nodular surface, features rarely seen in colonic tubular adenomas. The dysplastic epithelium of a polypoid sessile gastric adenoma typically occupies the upper portion of the mucosa while the subjacent non-neoplastic mucosa may remain unchanged or more often shows cystic dilatation of glands. The dysplastic epithelium of a flat or depressed adenoma occupies almost the entire thickness of the mucosa.

Tubular adenomas far outnumber villous or tubulovillous adenomas in the stomach. On the other hand, villous (papillary) and tubulovillous (papillotubular) patterns are more common in carcinoma than in adenoma of the stomach. The tubules of tubular adenoma are frequently unbranched. They are lined by crowded columnar cells with predominantly spindle-shaped and oval, homogeneously hyperchromatic nuclei with reduced or absent mucus. The nucleocytoplasmic ratio is usually 1:1. With increasing dysplasia the nuclei become wider, rounder, more hyperchromatic and stratified, and mitoses more numerous. When a dysplastic lesion consists of cells with large, round, vesicular nuclei containing dotted chromatin and distinct eosinophilic nucleoli, it may well represent a tubular adenocarcinoma.

The majority of gastric adenomas have epithelium showing intestinal features, i. e. intestinal absorptive-type cells with or without brush borders, goblet cells, Paneth cells and intestinal-type endocrine cells. A proportion may have mixed varieties of epithelium with both intestinal and gastric foveolar features. Adenomas of pyloric gland type akin to those of the gallbladder are extremely rare in the stomach.

The size of gastric adenoma is under 2 cm in about 80%-90% of cases. The frequency of its malignant transformation depends largely on the size; up to 2% in adenomas under 2 cm and 40%-50% in adenomas larger than 2 cm.

1.2 Malignant

1.2.1 Adenocarcinoma

A malignant tumour of glandular epithelium composed of tubular, acinar, or papillary structures.

Most carcinomas of the stomach are adenocarcinomas. The tumour cells may resemble either intestinal or gastric epithelium in their structure and function. Variable numbers of Paneth cells or endocrine cells may be present. They are frequently seen in the deep mucosal layer of the tumour. In addition, there may be scattered parietal cells or α-fetoprotein secreting cells. However the presence of these specialized elements does not alter the classification.

Variation in the histological type and degree of cell differentiation in different parts of a gastric adenocarcinoma is often very striking and much greater than in the colon. In the diagnosis of gastric adenocarcinoma it is recommended that typing be based on the predominant feature, with the minor components referred to in the description.

1.2.1.1 Papillary Adenocarcinoma (Figs. 43–47)
An adenocarcinoma composed of pointed or blunt finger-like epithelial processes with fibrovascular cores.

The tumour cells are cylindrical or cuboidal and usually maintain a well-polarized surface orientation. In some tumours there may be a severe degree of cellular and nuclear pleomorphism. The papillary subtype may show tubular differentiation (papillotubular).

Papillary adenocarcinoma typically grows as a polypoid mass projecting into the gastric lumen. When deep invasion occurs, peripheral demarcation is often sharp, and there may be infiltration by acute and chronic inflammatory cells.

1.2.1.2 Tubular Adenocarcinoma (Figs. 48–61)
An adenocarcinoma composed predominantly of branching tubules embedded in or surrounded by fibrous stroma.

The cross-sectional diameter of the tubules varies, and there can be cystic dilatation. The tumour cells are cylindrical or cuboidal but may be flattened by the accumulation of luminal mucin. Adenocarcinomas with both acinar (glandular) and solid structures as well as adenocarcinoma with lymphoid stroma are included in this category.

1.2.1.3 Mucinous Adenocarcinoma (Figs. 62, 63)
An adenocarcinoma in which a substantial amount of extracellular mucin (more than 50% of the tumour) is retained within the tumour.

The mucin can usually be observed macroscopically. Two growth patterns are encountered: (a) glands lined by a columnar mucous-secreting epithelium together with interstitial mucin (well-differentiated type), and (b) chains or irregular clusters of cells surrounded by mucus (poorly differentiated type). Some tumours show both growth patterns. Signet-ring cells may be present. However more than 50% of a tumour should comprise signet-ring cells before it is classified as signet-ring cell carcinoma.

Mucinous adenocarcinomas composed of cells in small irregular clusters or containing significant numbers of signet-ring cells may be graded as poorly differentiated. However grading becomes unreliable when there is excessive mucus and only a few cellular elements remain.

The term mucinous adenocarcinoma is used synonymously with mucoid, colloid and muconodular adenocarcinoma.

1.2.1.4 Signet-ring Cell Carcinoma (Figs. 64–68)

An adenocarcinoma in which a predominant component (more than 50% of the tumour) is made up of isolated or small-groups of malignant cells containing intracytoplasmic mucin.

Typically the volume of intracytoplasmic mucin is sufficient to compress the nucleus against the periphery of the cell, giving the classical signet-ring appearance. The amount of intracytoplasmic mucin varies from cell to cell. Four types of tumour cells are encountered: (a) those with an intracytoplasmic cyst filled with acid mucin; (b) those distended with secretory granules of acid or neutral mucin; (c) elements with eosinophilic cytoplasmic granules containing neutral mucin; and (d) cells without mucin. These cell types may occur independently or in combination within any one tumour.

Although signet-ring cells do not form tubules, they are functionally glandular, and there is often an admixed glandular component particularly in the deep mucosa of intramucosal signet-ring cell carcinoma. Thus it is appropriate to classify signet-ring cell tumours under adenocarcinoma.

In the mucosa of some cases, especially early carcinomas, signet-ring cell carcinoma shows a three-layered pattern; the upper-most layer contains signet-ring cells with mucin of gastric surface epithelial type; the middle layer, cells without mucin; and the lowest layer, cells with mucin of pyloric glandular epithelial type. Such an organized differentiation in the tumour, as seen in the normal mucosa, is not found in regions other than the mucosa. In the deep layers of the gastric wall, signet-ring cell carcinoma often has many non-mucous containing cells.

Signet-ring cells tend to infiltrate diffusely and may be associated with considerable fibrosis (scirrhous carcinoma). Such carcinomas may involve the entire stomach and have been described as linitis plastica. Here the malignant nature of the condition may be obscured by fibrosis. Stains for mucin or the immunohistochemical demonstration of cytokeratin should clarify diagnostic problems.

A number of conditions may mimic signet-ring cell carcinoma. The presence of lipid or mucin-containing macrophages within the lamina propria of non-specific gastritis, the gastritis due to bile reflux or pancreatitis must be differentiated from intramucosal signet-ring cell carcinoma. Macrophage nuclei are typically regular and are more centrally located than signet-ring cell nuclei. Detached and degenerating epithelial cells may round up and simulate signet-ring cells in active gastritis. Lymphoid cells may become distended with immunoglobulin in the rare so-called signet-ring cell lymphoma.

Signet-ring cell carcinoma is synonymous with mucocellular carcinoma.

* *
*

Adenocarcinoma of the stomach may be graded in the following manner:

Well-differentiated: an adenocarcinoma with a regular glandular structure that often closely resembles metaplastic intestinal epithelium.
Moderately differentiated: an adenocarcinoma intermediate between well differentiated and poorly differentiated.
Poorly differentiated: an adenocarcinoma composed either of highly irregular glands that are recognized with difficulty or of single cells or cells in small or large solid clusters with mucus-secreting cells or acinar (glandular) structures.

Adenocarcinoma may also be graded as low grade (well or moderately differentiated) or high grade (poorly differentiated).

* *
*

The following terms are used to describe growth patterns or stromal reactions in gastric carcinomas:

Solid: the cells are closely packed and the tumours have a well-defined boundary. They may either be undifferentiated (undifferentiated carcinoma, small cell carcinoma) or contain glandular structures or mucus-secreting cells (poorly differentiated adenocarcinoma).
Scirrhous: the tumour cells are few relative to the fibrous stroma. This pattern is characteristic of "linitis plastica" but may not be reproduced in metastatic deposits.
Lymphoid stroma: the entire tumour tissue is diffusely infiltrated by lymphoid cells, predominantly lymphocytes and plasma cells, with occasional lymphoid follicles. The histological type of the tumour is mainly a poorly differentiated tubular adenocarcinoma. The frequency of carcinoma with lymphoid stroma is about 4% of gastric carcinomas.

Superficial spreading carcinoma: extensive lateral spread of the tumour, primarily in the mucosa and superficial submucosa. It is not synonymous with intramucosal carcinoma.
Carcinoma in situ: adenocarcinoma which has not invaded the lamina propria (Sect. 8). This diagnosis may be difficult or impossible to make with certainty especially on endoscopic biopsy.
Intramucosal carcinoma: carcinoma has spread within the lamina propria but not beyond the muscularis mucosae. Lymph node metastasis is found in about 2%-3% of the cases.

1.2.2 Adenosquamous Carcinoma (Fig. 69)

A single tumour in which both adenocarcinomatous and squamous carcinomatous components are present.

This is distinct from adenocarcinoma with small foci of squamous metaplasia which should be classified under adenocarcinoma, with the squamous components referred to in the description. A tumour with a distinct boundary between both components in the same mass may or may not be a collision tumour and may be tentatively included in this type.

1.2.3 Squamous Cell Carcinoma (Fig. 70)

A malignant epithelial tumour composed of cells resembling those of squamous epithelium.

In the majority of cases reported as gastric squamous cell carcinoma, small foci of adenocarcinoma have been found. Most squamous cell carcinomas of the cardia are the result of spread from a tumour in the oesophagus.

1.2.4 Small Cell Carcinoma (Figs. 71-76)

A malignant tumour similar in histology, histochemistry, ultrastructure and clinical behaviour to small cell carcinoma of the lung.

This tumour has a solid or sheet-like structure with occasional acinar patterns and vascular stroma. The cytoplasm is scant or eosinophilic granular. The nuclei are round or oval and fairly uniform in size and shape, and they are usually larger than those of a gastric carcinoid tumour. The chromatin is fine and diffusely distributed, and nucleoli are indistinct or small and basophilic. There are frequent mitotic figures. Many of the tumour cells contain argyrophil (Grimelius-positive) granules or dense-core granules (electron microscopically) in their cytoplasm. These granules may be positive for serotonin, peptide YY, somatostatin and gastrin, but positive cells are not frequent. The tumour has been called endocrine cell carcinoma and neuroendocrine carcinoma. Its frequency is about 0.6% of all malignant epithelial tumours of the stomach.

The tumour usually contains an adenocarcinomatous component especially in the mucosa, which often disappears due to ulceration in advanced cases. Small cell carcinoma with adenocarcinoma has been called adeno-endocrine cell carcinoma or adeno-small cell carcinoma and probably accounts for almost all of the so-called mixed carcinoid-adenocarcinomas reported in the literature. The term mixed carcinoid-adenocarcinoma should be reserved for a tumour with classical carcinoid and adenocarcinoma (Sect. 2.2).

1.2.5 Undifferentiated Carcinoma (Fig. 77)

A malignant epithelial tumour that has no glandular structure or other features to indicate definite differentiation.

Terms such as carcinoma simplex, carcinoma solidum and medullary carcinoma were used in earlier times for these tumours. Undifferentiated carcinoma may be distinguished from poorly differentiated adenocarcinoma, small cell carcinoma (oat cell carcinoma), lymphoma and leukaemic deposits by the use of mucin stains, argyrophil techniques for neuroendocrine granules or immunohistochemical methods.

1.2.6 Others

Primary gastric choriocarcinoma (Figs. 78, 79) and embryonal carcinoma have been described. They usually have an adenocarcinomatous component.

* *
*

Classification of Laurén

In addition to the traditional classification given above, gastric carcinoma may also be subdivided into intestinal and diffuse types. This distinction has been found to be particularly useful in epidemiological studies.

The *intestinal type* is typically characterized by a predominance of glandular epithelium that often includes tall, intestinal-type columnar cells with brush borders and goblet cells secreting acid mucins. In addition, and as in incomplete types of intestinal metaplasia, the columnar cells may contain apically located mucin which is usually sulphated. The cells may also show clear cell differentiation. Intestinal metaplastic mucosa is often widespread in the vicinity of the tumour. The neoplasm is typically well circumscribed with a pushing margin. There may be a well-developed peritumoural lymphocytic infiltrate.

The *diffuse type* of carcinoma may show, particularly in the surface of the superficial part of the tumour, some glandular arrangements but is mainly characterized by poorly cohesive, rather small rounded cells with wide and diffuse infiltration of the gastric wall. The tumour is poorly demarcated. Many of the cells contain mucus and can show the typical signet-ring cell shape, but non-secreting cells occur also. As in intestinal carcinomas, the mucins include acidic and neutral sugars. However there is usually little or no sulphation of mucus.

Paneth cells and endocrine cells as well as interstitial mucus may be present in both intestinal and diffuse types.

Whereas the majority of gastric carcinomas can be subdivided into intestinal and diffuse types, a minority cannot be so classified. These include tumours with about equal proportions of intestinal and diffuse characteristics and others that are undifferentiated and have a solid growth pattern. These are placed into an *indeterminate* category. Squamous cell carcinoma and adenosquamous carcinoma are categorized separately.

Classification of Ming

This divides gastric carcinoma into two types - expanding and infiltrating. The term *expanding* encompasses carcinomas that are relatively well circumscribed with a pushing growth margin whereas *infiltrating* types are diffusely spreading growths. These categories are roughly similar to the intestinal and diffuse types of Laurén. However, not only is it possible to classify the great majority of gastric carcinomas as expanding or infiltrating, but Ming's system has the merit of simplicity and clinical relevance. Thus a greater margin of surgical clearance would be required for infiltrating cancers.

Some carcinomas may include both intestinal/expanding and diffuse/infiltrating components. Classifications can be slanted either histogenetically, epidemiologically or clinically. From the clinical standpoint, the classification should be based on the least favourable area whereas the most well differentiated component could provide useful histogenetic or epidemiological information.

2 Endocrine Tumours

2.1 Carcinoid Tumour (Figs. 80-82)

Carcinoid tumours arise from the basal part of the gastric mucosa where endocrine cells are most numerous. They occur more frequently in the body than in the antrum of the stomach. They tend to infiltrate the submucosa early, often appearing as a submucosal tumour. The overlying mucosa may be elevated, atrophic, eroded, or ulcerated. Carcinoid tumours are composed of uniform cells of small to medium size with abundant eosinophilic granular cytoplasm and poorly defined cell boundaries. The cells are arranged in solid, trabecular or anastomosing trabecular structures and sometimes in rosettes or acini. They have round to oval regular nuclei and no or exceedingly rare mitotic figures.

On electron microscopy the cytoplasm contains characteristic dense-core granules. These granules are argyrophil (e.g. by the Bodian, Grimelius or lead haematoxylin methods), less frequently argentaffin (e.g. by the Fontana-Masson method) or non-reactive. Immunohistochemical techniques may demonstrate the endocrine nature of the tumour cells through the identification of specific markers (e.g. chromogranin), amines (e.g. serotonin) and polypeptides (e.g. gastrin, somatostatin, peptide YY). Positive cells are, however, not plentiful in general.

Carcinoid tumours are rare in the stomach comprising approximately 0.4% of malignant gastric epithelial tumours. The majority behave in a low-grade malignant manner. A proportion arises within a background of diffuse endocrine cell hyperplasia (intraglandular proliferation) and multiple endocrine cell micronests (extraglandular proliferation) in patients with achlorhydria and hypergastrinaemia, e.g. in pernicious anaemia or type A gastritis.

The term *microcarcinoidosis* (Fig. 81) has been applied to multiple, small (less than 5 mm) collections of endocrine cells not forming a distinct tumour. This may represent a variant of diffuse endocrine cell hyperplasia and multiple endocrine cell micronests in patients with pernicious anaemia, type A gastritis or gastrinoma (Sect. 7.7).

2.2 Mixed Carcinoid-Adenocarcinoma

A tumour with clear-cut adenocarcinomatous and classical carcinoid components.

These are very rare in the stomach. A proportion of adenocarcinomas contain scattered endocrine elements. Such tumours should be classified as adenocarcinomas. A tumour with adenocarcinoma and small cell carcinoma should be classified under small cell carcinoma because of its aggressive behaviour clinically (Sect. 1.2.4).

3 Non-epithelial Tumours

See *Histological Typing of Soft Tissue Tumours* for definitions and explanatory notes

3.1 Benign

3.1.1 Leiomyoma (Fig. 83)

This is the most common non-epithelial tumour of the stomach. Typical histological features are interlacing bundles of uniform eosinophilic spindle-shaped cells surrounded by reticulin fibres and containing elongated nuclei with blunt ends. Mitotic figures are absent or very sparse. Leiomyomas may become fibrotic and calcified. Commonly they are small (less than 2 cm in diameter) and can be multiple. They arise from muscle of the cardia, fornix and body of the stomach. They may be intramural, but larger tumours protrude from the outer or inner surface of the stomach (or both, dumbbell-shaped). Ulceration is common in larger growths. Tumours with prominent nuclear palisading may simulate neurilemmomas. Occasionally the distinction from neurilemmoma is difficult but may be facilitated by means of immunohistochemistry, especially in respect to S100 protein which is present in neurogenic tumours and absent in smooth muscle tumours. Desmin may not be demonstrable in smooth muscle tumours of the stomach and intestines. The generic term stromal tumour has been used for tumours not clearly of muscle or neural type.

Leiomyomas may be composed wholly or partly of rounded or polygonal cells with a clear space partially or completely surrounding the nucleus or with acidophilic cytoplasm. The clear space is an artefact and does not appear in well-fixed specimens. Smooth muscle tumours comprising such cells have been described as *epithelioid leiomyoma* or *leiomyoblastoma* (Fig. 84).

3.1.2 Lipoma

3.1.3 Vascular Tumours

3.1.3.1 Haemangioma

3.1.3.2 Lymphangioma

3.1.3.3 Glomus Tumour (Fig. 85)

This usually occurs in the muscle coat of the gastric wall. It contains epithelioid cells with uniform round nuclei, sharply defined cell borders and prominent vascular spaces.

3.1.4 Neurogenic Tumours

These resemble their counterparts outside the gastrointestinal tract. They are typically positive for S100 protein immunohistochemically.

3.1.4.1 Neurilemmoma (Schwannoma) (Figs. 86, 87)

3.1.4.2 Neurofibroma

3.1.4.3 Granular Cell Tumour

This usually occurs in the submucosa.

3.1.5 Others

3.2 Malignant

3.2.1 Leiomyosarcoma (Fig. 88)

This is the most common malignant soft tissue tumour of the stomach. It can be vascular, haemorrhagic, necrotic, cystic and ulcerated, and so its appearance is frequently altered by these changes. The tumour may present as a large cystic mass within the abdominal cavity, connected to the wall of the stomach by a narrow pedicle. The distinction between leiomyosarcoma and leiomyoma may be difficult. The most important single criterion for malignancy is the number of mitotic figures. Counts in excess of ten per 50 high-power fields are usually indicative of malignancy. Other features are large tumour size (over 5 cm), necrosis, invasion of adjacent tissues and organs, dense cellularity and a high nucleocytoplasmic ratio. However it is often difficult to predict the behaviour of smooth muscle tumours in individual patients. Epithelioid features as described in leiomyomas may be present in leiomyosarcomas (Sect. 3.1.1).

3.2.2 Kaposi Sarcoma

3.2.3 Malignant Neurilemmoma (Malignant Schwannoma, Neurogenic Sarcoma)

3.2.4 Others

4 Malignant Lymphoma

Lymphomas can be primary or secondary. Primary gastric lymphoma may be single, multiple or widely diffused. Single tumours may form nodular or polypoid masses which usually ulcerate. Diffuse lymphoma may give rise to a mixture of swelling and multiple shallow depressions of the mucosa or a cerebriform rugal hypertrophy.

The classification of malignant lymphomas is far from standardized. However the Working Formulation and Kiel classification (presented in the table), which are widely used, can be applied to most gastrointestinal lymphomas and permit comparisons with other sites.

Gastrointestinal and nodal lymphomas may differ in certain respects. Gastrointestinal lymphomas often show considerable pleomorphism and may contain a mixture of reactive cells. True follicular lymphoma (centroblastic-centrocytic) is very rare. However it should

Table. Working Formulation and Kiel Classification of non-Hodgkin lymphomas. From Cancer vol 49, p 2121, 1982

Working Formulation	Kiel equivalent or related terms
Low grade	
A. Malignant lymphoma	
Small lymphocytic	
Consistent with CLL	ML lymphocytic, CLL
Plasmacytoid	ML lymphoplasmacytic/lymphoplasmacytoid
B. Malignant lymphoma, follicular Predominantly small cleaved cell Diffuse areas Sclerosis C. Malignant lymphoma, follicular Mixed small cleaved and large cell Diffuse areas Sclerosis	ML centroblastic-centrocytic (small), follicular ± diffuse

Table (continued)

Working Formulation	Kiel equivalent or related terms
Intermediate grade	
D. Malignant lymphoma, follicular	ML centroblastic-centrocytic (large),
Predominantly large cell	follicular ± diffuse
Diffuse areas	
Sclerosis	
E. Malignant lymphoma, diffuse	ML centrocytic (small)
Small cleaved cell	
Sclerosis	
F. Malignant lymphoma, diffuse	ML centroblastic-centrocytic (small),
Mixed small and large cell	diffuse
Sclerosis	ML lymphoplasmacytic/-cytoid,
Epithelioid cell component	polymorphic
G. Malignant lymphoma, diffuse	
Large cell	ML centroblastic-centrocytic (large),
Cleaved cell	diffuse
Noncleaved cell	ML centrocytic (large)
Sclerosis	ML centroblastic
High grade	
H. Malignant lymphoma	
Large cell, immunoblastic	ML immunoblastic
Plasmacytoid	
Clear cell	
Polymorphous	T-zone lymphoma
Epithelioid cell component	Lymphoepithelioid cell lymphoma
I. Malignant lymphoma	
Lymphoblastic	
Convoluted cell	ML lymphoblastic, convoluted cell
Nonconvoluted cell	ML lymphoblastic, unclassified
J. Malignant lymphoma	
Small noncleaved cell	
Burkitt's	ML lymphoblastic, Burkitt type and
Follicular areas	other B-lymphoblastic
Miscellaneous	
Composite	-
Mycosis fungoides	Mycosis fungoides
Histiocytic	-
Extramedullary plasmacytoma	ML plasmacytic
Unclassifiable	-
Other	-

CLL, chronic lymphocytic leukaemia; ML, malignant lymphoma

be appreciated that reactive lymphoid follicles are frequently seen in B-cell lymphomas. These may be invaded or surrounded by neoplastic lymphoid cells. Nodular aggregates may be formed by some diffuse lymphomas, notably in lymphomatous polyposis. Plasma cell differentiation should be recorded; the immunohistochemical demonstration of light-chain restriction provides important evidence of monoclonality. Primary Hodgkin disease and true histiocytic lymphoma of the stomach are vanishingly rare.

The distinction between a tumour-like mass of benign lymphoid hyperplasia (pseudolymphoma) and low-grade B-cell lymphoma may pose diagnostic difficulties. Some speculate that these entities represent the two ends of a continuum in a single disease process. The demonstration of a monoclonal lymphoid population together with invasion and destruction of glandular epithelium by centrocyte-like cells (lymphoepithelial lesions) provides support for malignancy.

The following classification and commentary may serve as a useful supplement for gastrointestinal lymphoma.

4.1 B-Cell Lymphomas

4.1.1 Small Cell Lymphoma (Figs. 89–91)

A diffuse lymphoma in which at least 80% of cells are small lymphoid cells (small lymphocytes, plasma cells, lymphoplasmacytoid cells, centrocyte-like cells).

Lymphoid follicles are reactive, if present. Lymphoepithelial lesions (i. e. glands infiltrated and destroyed by lymphoid cells) may be seen (Fig. 91). Lymphoplasmacytoid cells may be distended with immunoglobulin, giving an appearance described as signet-ring cell lymphoma. This must be distingished from signet-ring cell carcinoma, for example, with antibodies to leukocyte common antigen, pan B- or pan T-antigens and cytokeratin or mucin studies.

4.1.2 Plasmacytoma (Figs. 92, 93)

This rarely occurs in the stomach.

4.1.3 Malignant Lymphomatous Polyposis

A diffuse lymphoma composed exclusively of centrocytes arranged in nodular or polypoid aggregates within the mucosa and submucosa.

The disease is rarely if ever limited to the stomach, involving long segments of the intestinal tract as well.

4.1.4 Follicular (Centroblastic-Centrocytic) Lymphoma (Fig. 94)

This occurs rarely in the stomach even though it is one of the commonest types of nodal lymphoma.

4.1.5 Large Cell Lymphoma (Fig. 95)

A diffuse and often polymorphic lymphoma in which at least 20% of cells are large lymphoid cells (centroblasts, immunoblasts).

Lymphoid follicles are reactive, if present. Lymphoepithelial lesions may be seen. Lymphomas composed exclusively of centroblasts or immunoblasts are uncommon. There is a rare variant of large cell or centroblastic lymphoma composed of cells with large multilobulated nuclei. This should be distinguished from T-cell lymphoma.

4.1.6 Burkitt-type (Lymphoblastic) Lymphoma

This occurs only rarely in the stomach.

4.2 T-Cell Lymphomas

These are rare in the stomach.

4.3 Unclassified Lymphoma

* *
*

Grading Lymphomas

Grading of lymphomas offers useful clinical guidance. The majority of low-grade lymphomas of the stomach are small B-cell lymphomas. Malignant lymphomatous polyposis has a slow but inexorable course and may be regarded as being of intermediate grade. High-grade lymphomas mainly comprise large B-cell tumours.

5 Miscellaneous Tumours

The very rare occurrence of teratoma, carcinosarcoma and malignant melanoma of the stomach has been described.

6 Secondary Tumours

7 Tumour-Like Lesions

7.1 Hyperplastic Polyp (Fig. 96)

A benign sessile or pedunculated polyp composed of irregular hyperplastic glands, the epithelium being mostly of the foveolar (i. e. superficial gastric) type, but pyloric (antral) glands, chief cells and parietal cells may be present; regenerative atypia in the epithelium (immature regenerating epithelium) and atypical reactive stromal cells may appear frequently after erosion.

Epithelial dysplasia or intramucosal adenocarcinoma is rare particularly in a polyp less than 2 cm in size, but there may be foci of intestinal metaplasia. Cystic change and superficial ulceration are common. The stroma may contain bands of fibromuscular tissue and show variable degrees of inflammatory cell infiltration and oedema.

Hyperplastic polyps can be single or multiple and are usually located in the antrum rather than in the body of the stomach. When multiple, they are often distributed along the boundary (transitional zone) of the antral and the fundic mucosa. They are common lesions and must be differentiated from the much less frequent adenoma, juvenile polyp, Cronkhite-Canada polyp and Peutz-Jeghers polyp.

Hyperplastic polyps have also been described as inflammatory polyps and regenerative polyps.

7.2 Hamartomas

7.2.1 Fundic Gland Polyp and Polyposis (Figs. 97-100)

A focal polypoid hyperplasia of fundic glands with variable degrees of foveolar and glandular cystic dilatation and with shortened foveolae.

These lesions usually present as multiple (usually less than 20) small polyps generally less than 5 mm in size in the body and fundus of the stomach (fundic mucosal area). They are not precancerous.

When hundreds of this type of gastric polyp are present, there is a strong association with familial adenomatosis coli.

7.2.2 **Peutz-Jeghers Polyp and Polyposis** (Figs. 101–103)

A lesion with excessive hyperplasia, elongation and cystic change of foveolar epithelium, reduced lamina propria and prominent cores of branching bands of smooth muscle derived from the muscularis mucosae, the deeper glandular components showing atrophy.

Gastric Peutz-Jeghers polyp is different in histology from the intestinal form, which is composed of a fairly balanced hyperplasia of the mucosa. Malignant change is uncommon especially in polyps less than 3 cm in size. Peutz-Jeghers polyps are usually multiple, as part of the syndrome of gastrointestinal polyposis.

7.2.3 **Juvenile Polyp and Polyposis** (Fig. 104)

Aggregated polypoid lesions characterized by irregular hyperplasia and cystic change of foveolae, with initially normal and later atrophic and cystic glands, separated from one another by an excess of oedematous superficial lamina propria, while the mucosa surrounding the polyps is essentially normal.

Although not conclusively established as a hamartomatous lesion it may be convenient to consider juvenile polyps under this heading. The lesions can be complicated by erosion and secondary infection leading to reactive hyperplasia of immature foveolar epithelium and formation of granulation tissue. It is usually multiple, as part of the syndrome of juvenile polyposis of the gastrointestinal tract. It should be distinguished from Peutz-Jeghers polyp, multiple isolated hyperplastic polyps and Cronkhite-Canada polyposis.

7.3 Heterotopias

7.3.1 **Pancreatic Heterotopia** (Fig. 105)

This is the most common variety of congenital heterotopia. When smooth muscle and ducts are the only components, the lesion has been described as adenomyoma or myoepithelial hamartoma.

7.3.2 **Gastric Gland Heterotopia** (Fig. 106)

This consists of gastric glandular elements with thin muscular bundles, and is predominantly located in the submucosa. Pyloric or pseudopyloric type glands are most common, associated with some fundic or intestinal type glands. Heterotopia of pure fundic or intestinal type glands is extremely rare. Gastric gland heterotopia may contain compact glands of pyloric type (so-called Brunner gland heterotopia) or show dilatation (gastritis cystica profunda or a submucosal cyst).

7.4 Hypertrophic Rugal Lesions

7.4.1 Giant Rugal Hypertrophy (Ménétrier Disease) (Figs. 107–109)

Thickened fundic type mucosa, initially with balanced mucosal hyperplasia and later with fundic gland atrophy, pseudopyloric gland metaplasia (or mucous neck cell hyperplasia), cystic change in the deep mucosa and relative elongation of foveolae and finally with widening of superficial lamina propria and erosion.

These changes occur in a diffuse or a localized form. This should be distinguished from other hypertrophic rugal lesions or superficial gastritis with severe inflammatory infiltrates of the fundic mucosa.

7.4.2 Fundic Gland Hyperplasia (Zollinger-Ellison Syndrome)

Thickened fundic mucosa due to hyperplasia of parietal, chief and endocrine cells with shortened foveolae.

This occurs in the Zollinger-Ellison syndrome due to trophic action of increased serum gastrin secreted by a gastrinoma or G cell hyperplasia.

7.4.3 Gastritis Cystica Polyposa (Stomal Polypoid Hypertrophic Gastritis) (Figs. 110, 111)

Thickened mucosa or sessile polypoid lesions of the gastric mucosa at and near an anastomotic site, characterized by hyperplasia of immature and mature foveolar epithelium, florid cystic change, pseudopyloric gland metaplasia and atrophy of fundic glands accompanied by displacement of cystic epithelium into the submucosa.

This occurs at and near a gastrojejunal or gastroduodenal anastomosis. It begins as a stomal gastritis which later forms a localized or diffuse (circular) thickening of mucosal folds. This may prolapse and/or result in the formation of a polyp or mass which should be distinguished from a well-differentiated tubular or mucinous adenocarcinoma.

7.5 **Cronkhite-Canada Polyposis** (Figs. 112, 113)

Oedematous expansion of the lamina propria, hyperplasia and cystic change of foveolae and subsequent atrophy of glands leading to a diffuse swelling of the mucosa and multiple sessile polyps occurring in both the pyloric and the fundic mucosa.

Patients have gastrointestinal polyposis in general as well as a protein-losing enteropathy, alopecia, nail atrophy and skin pigmentation. Cases treated medically often show a decrease in the amount of oedema. There are a few cases of Cronkhite-Canada polyposis limited to the stomach, which usually have hypoproteinaemia due to the protein-losing gastropathy.

7.6 **Inflammatory Fibroid Polyp** (Figs. 114, 115)

A circumscribed polypoid lesion composed of a background of fibroblasts and blood vessels, infiltrated by a variable number of, but sometimes numerous, eosinophils, the blood vessels being typically surrounded by fibroblasts arranged in an onion-skin pattern.

The lesion is usually present in the pyloric mucosa, well demarcated and found mainly in the submucosa and the basal portion of the mucosa. It may extend partially into the muscle coat. Subsequent ulceration may occur especially over a large polyp.

The lesion is unrelated to histiocytosis X, eosinophilic gastritis and other allergic diseases, and the foreign body granulomatous reaction associated with certain parasites and food material.

7.7 **Endocrine Cell Hyperplasia and Micronest** (Figs. 116, 117)

Endocrine cells may increase in number in the gastric glands (endocrine cell hyperplasia) or be present in the lamina propria and/or muscularis mucosae (endocrine cell micronest) in non-specific or specific gastritis. In non-specific gastritis, the endocrine cells are composed mainly of a combination of gastrin-, serotonin- and somatostatin-producing cells. However, in patients with hypergastrinaemia, for example, in pernicious anaemia and type A gastritis, the cells are exclusively enterochromaffin-like cells (Sect. 2.1).

7.8 Benign Lymphoid Hyperplasia (Figs. 118, 119)

A lesion in which there is a reactive type of lymphoid hyperplasia.

The lesion may be diffuse or localized and can produce an ill-defined swelling of mucosa with erosions and/or ulceration. There is a marked proliferation of well-defined lymphoid follicles with germinal centres in the mucosa and submucosa, and even in the deeper layers of the gastric wall. Infiltration by a mixture of lymphocytes, plasma cells, eosinophils and histiocytes is seen between the follicles. There may be associated ulceration and fibrosis. Absence of atypia of the lymphoid cells, presence of well-defined follicles, a mixture of various inflammatory cells, and a polyclonal lymphoid cell population by immunohistochemistry characterize the benign reactive nature of the lesion.

7.9 Others

This category includes anisakiasis (acute form, with eosinophilic gastritis; chronic form, granulomatous; Fig. 120), malakoplakia, chronic peptic ulcer with abundant fibrous tissue, tuberculosis, sarcoidosis, syphilis, giant rugal lesion due to inflammatory extension of pancreatitis and xanthogranulomatous cholecystitis.

8 Epithelial Abnormalities (Precancerous)

8.1 Dysplasia

Atypical changes in the epithelium considered to be precancerous.

These include cytological abnormalities such as nuclear enlargement, hyperbasophilia, polarity-loss and pseudostratification, as well as changes in the architectural arrangement of glands, such as irregular branching, budding and complex growth patterns, all falling short of carcinoma in situ.

This occurs mainly in the intestinalized epithelium associated with chronic atrophic gastritis but may also develop within non-metaplastic gastric mucosa. Dysplasia is graded by its degree of severity into mild, moderate or severe, the first two being equivalent to low-grade and the last, high-grade dysplasia. Dysplasia is the most reliable marker for assessing the risk of adenocarcinoma, especially of the intestinal type.

Usually the histological findings of low-grade dysplasia are similar to those of adenoma. The distinction between severe dysplasia and carcinoma in situ or intramucosal adenocarcinoma can be difficult. A complex growth pattern with cribriform structure or a pattern with multiple glands without intervening stroma (back-to-back glands) or dysplastic tubules showing marked nuclear pseudostratification and enlarged, round to oval nuclei or dysplastic tubules having large, round vesicular nuclei with dotted chromatin and distinct eosinophilic nucleoli are the features generally favouring carcinoma in situ or intramucosal adenocarcinoma.

Reactive and regenerative changes in gastrointestinal epithelium differ in a number of respect from dysplasia. They show a gradual transition of epithelial atypicality to the lateral and subjacent surrounding epithelium (no front formation), uniform enlargement of nuclei with homogeneous basophilia, smooth margin and well-preserved polarity, regular arrangement with no high density of tubules, and widened inflamed vascular stroma. It may sometimes be difficult on biopsy to make a distinction between dysplasia and immature regenerative epithelium at the edges of an ulcer, an erosion and an eroded hyperplastic polyp.

Dysplasia may on occasion be found in hyperplastic polyps, Peutz-Jeghers polyps and juvenile polyposis.

Subject Index

Unless otherwise stated, all the preparations shown in the photomicrographs reproduced on the following pages were stained with haematoxylin-eosin.

×30

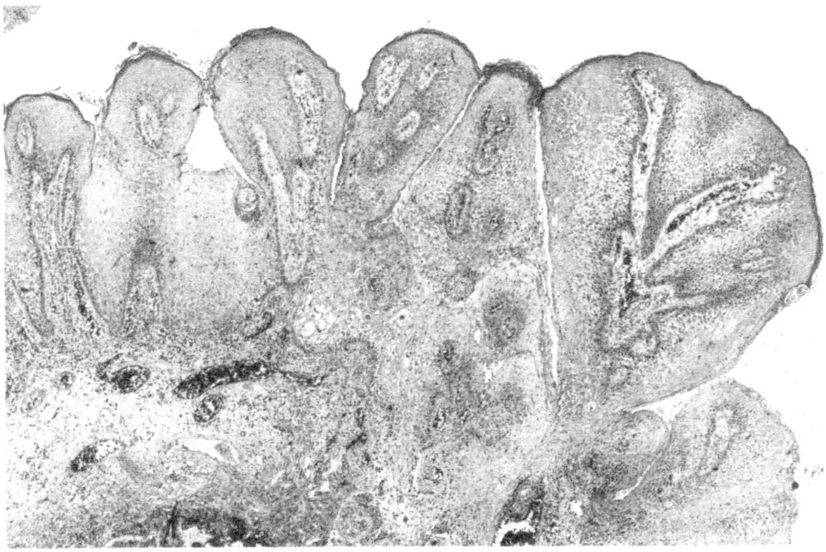

Fig. 1. *Squamous cell papilloma, oesophagus.* Polypectomy specimen

×150

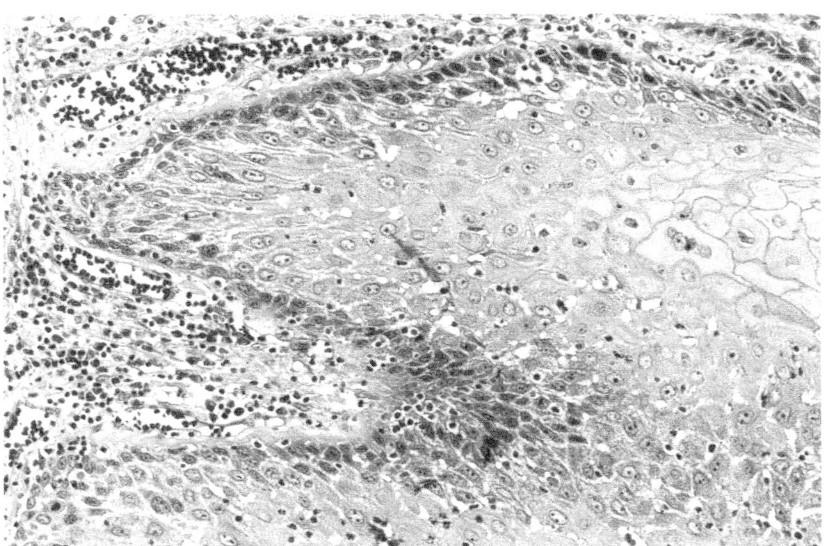

Fig. 2. *Squamous cell papilloma, oesophagus.* Same case as Fig. 1

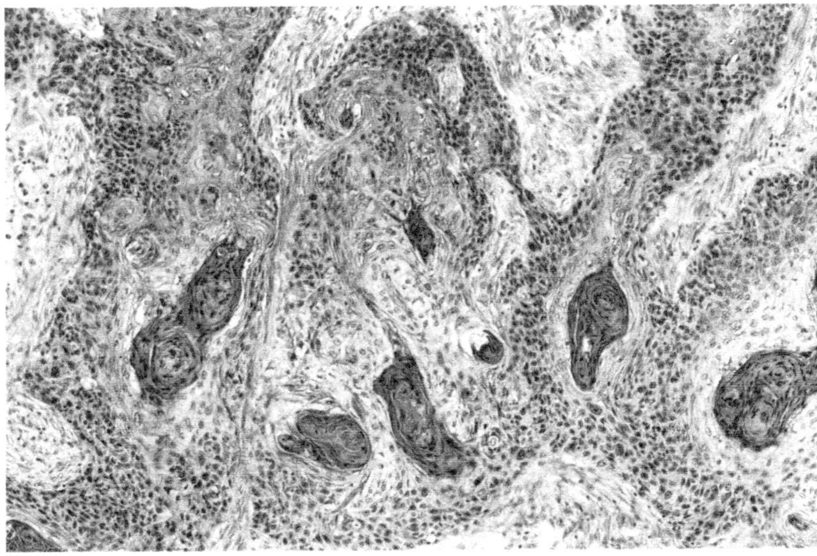

×75

Fig. 3. *Squamous cell carcinoma, oesophagus.* Well differentiated

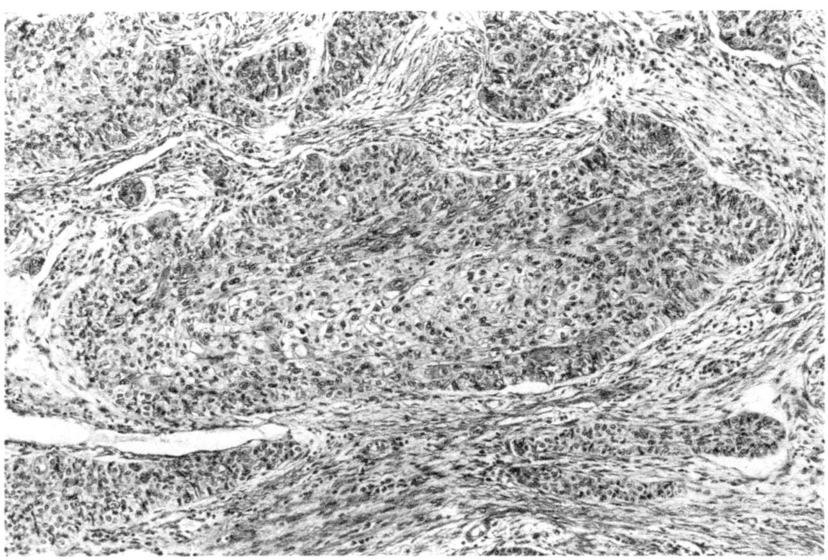

×75

Fig. 4. *Squamous cell carcinoma, oesophagus.* Moderately differentiated

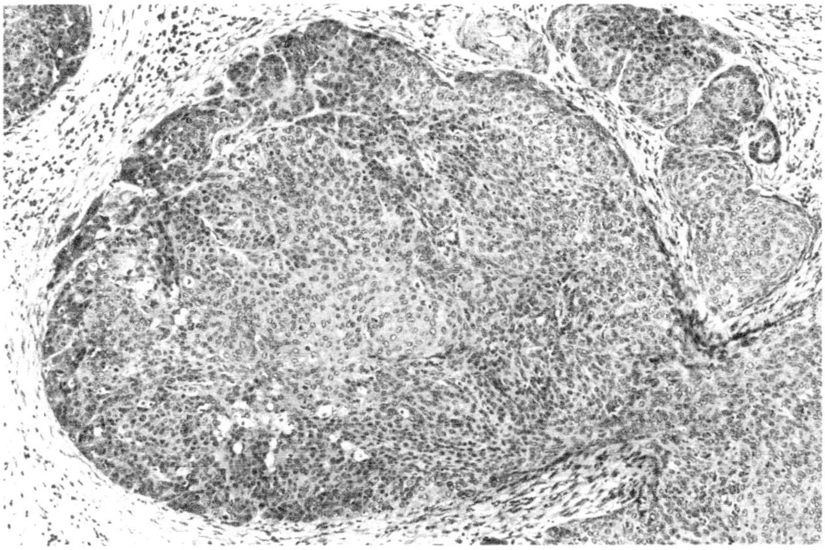

×75

Fig. 5. *Squamous cell carcinoma, oesophagus.* Moderately differentiated

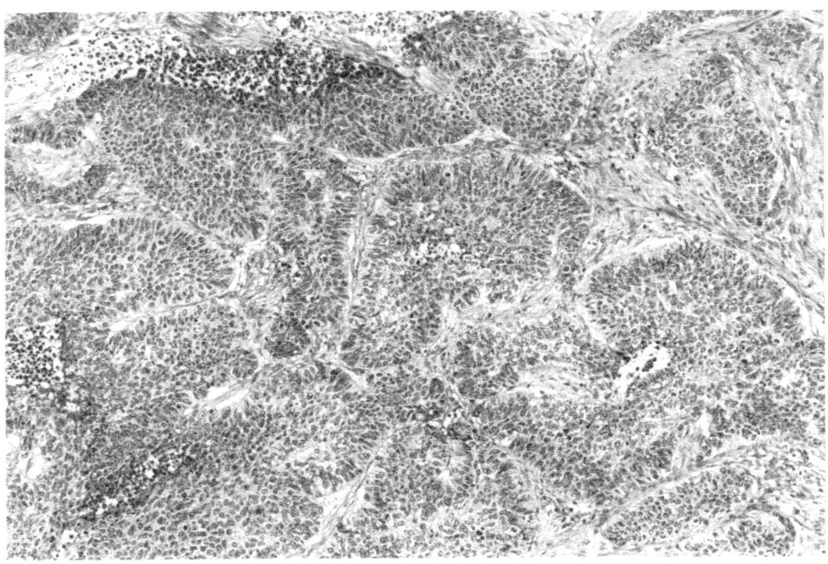

×75

Fig. 6. *Squamous cell carcinoma, oesophagus.* Poorly differentiated

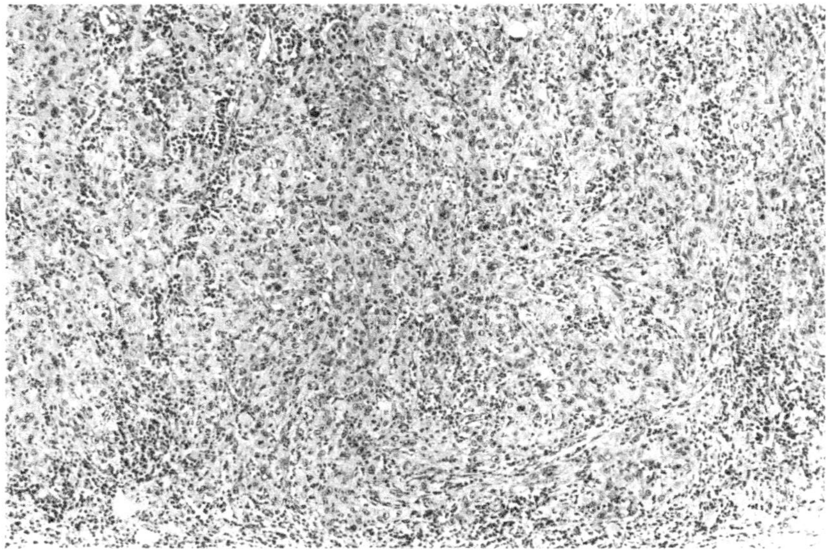

× 75

Fig. 7. *Squamous cell carcinoma, oesophagus.* Poorly differentiated

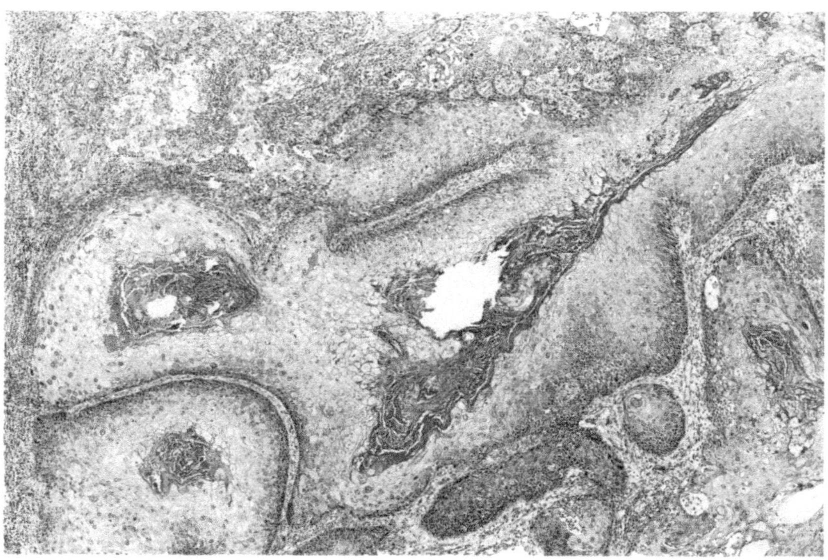

× 30

Fig. 8. *Verrucous (squamous) carcinoma, oesophagus.* Luminal surface at the right

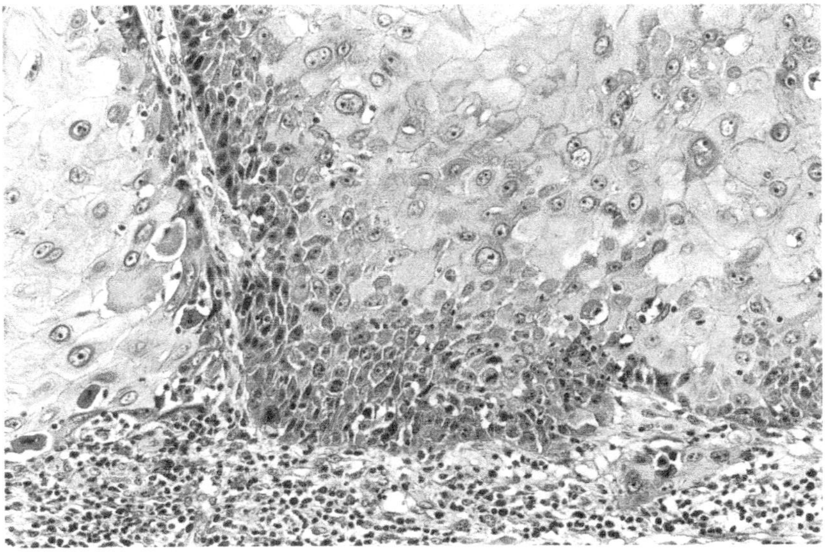

× 150

Fig. 9. *Verrucous (squamous) carcinoma, oesophagus.* Magnification of advancing margin of left lower corner of Fig. 8

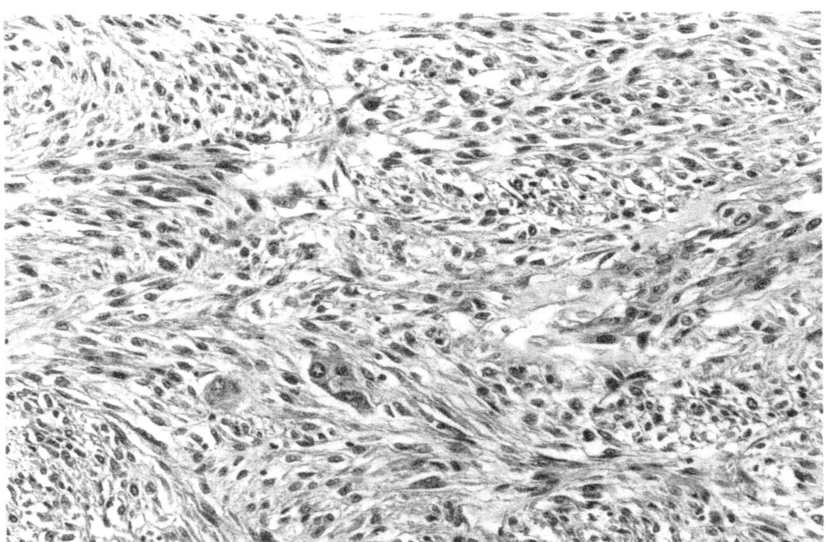

× 150

Fig. 10. *Spindle cell (squamous) carcinoma, oesophagus.* Small epithelial nests

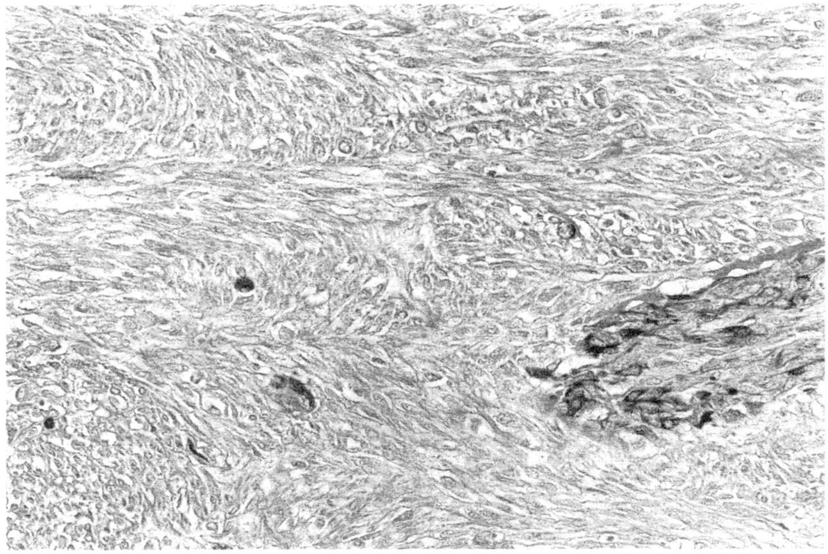

× 150

Fig. 11. *Spindle cell (squamous) carcinoma, oesophagus.* Keratin immunostaining positive in a few spindle cells and cells in epithelial nests. Same case as Fig. 10

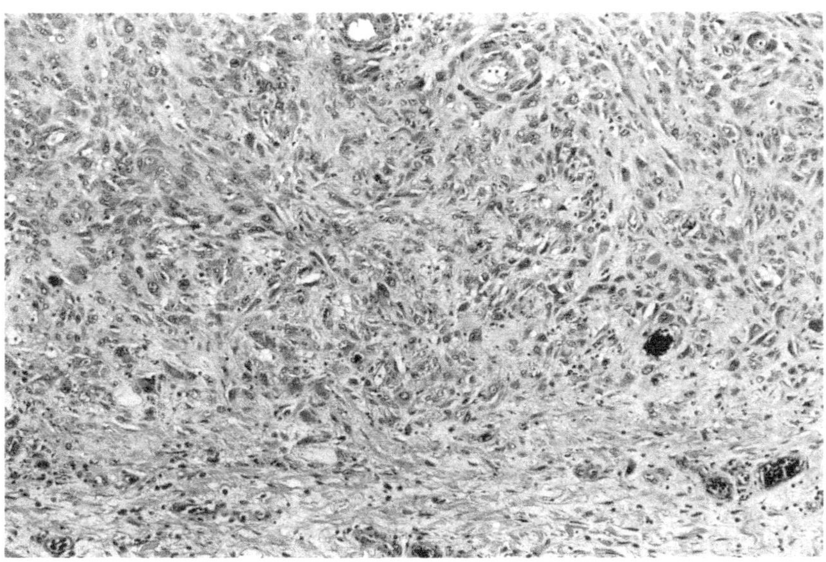

× 75

Fig. 12. *Spindle cell (squamous) carcinoma, oesophagus.* Advancing margin of polypoid tumour

× 75

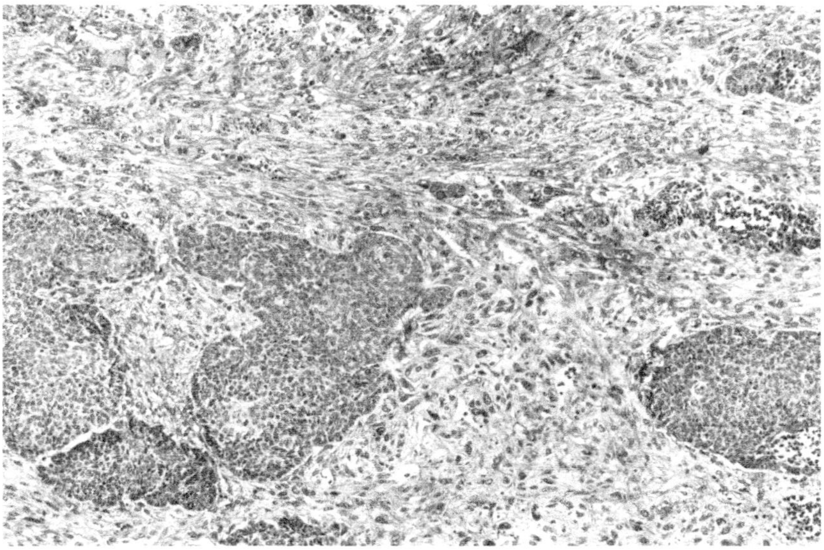

Fig. 13. *Spindle cell (squamous) carcinoma, oesophagus.* Islands of squamous cells embedded in sarcomatous stroma

× 30

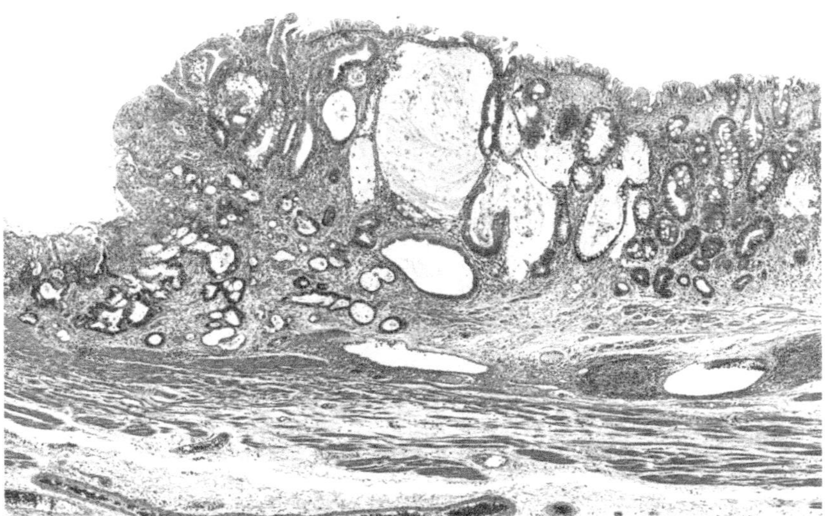

Fig. 14. *Adenocarcinoma in Barrett oesophagus.* Moderately differentiated tubular. Severe intestinal metaplasia in adjacent mucosa

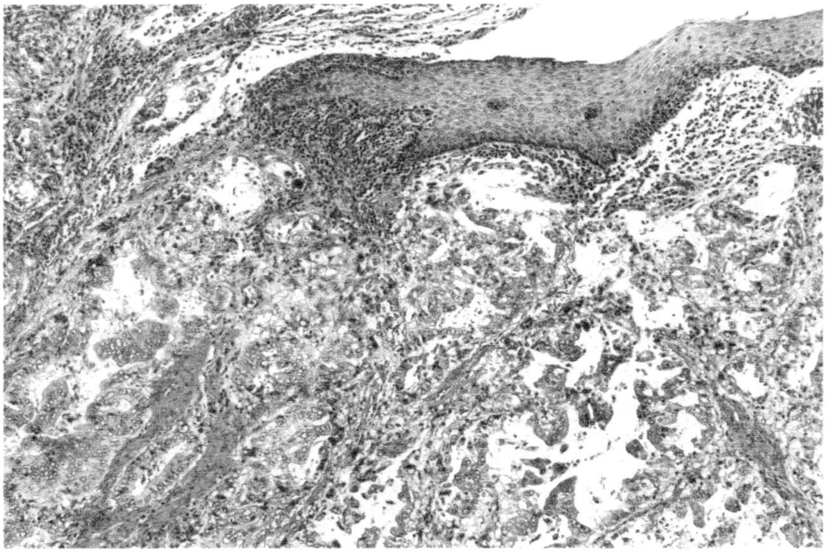

× 75

Fig. 15. *Adenocarcinoma, oesophagus.* Papillotubular adenocarcinoma in cervical oesophagus

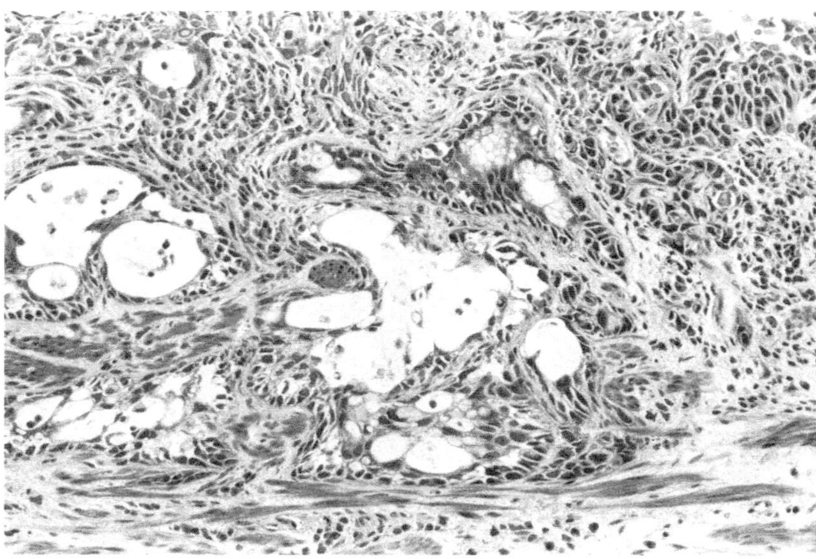

× 150

Fig. 16. *Mucoepidermoid carcinoma, oesophagus*

×300

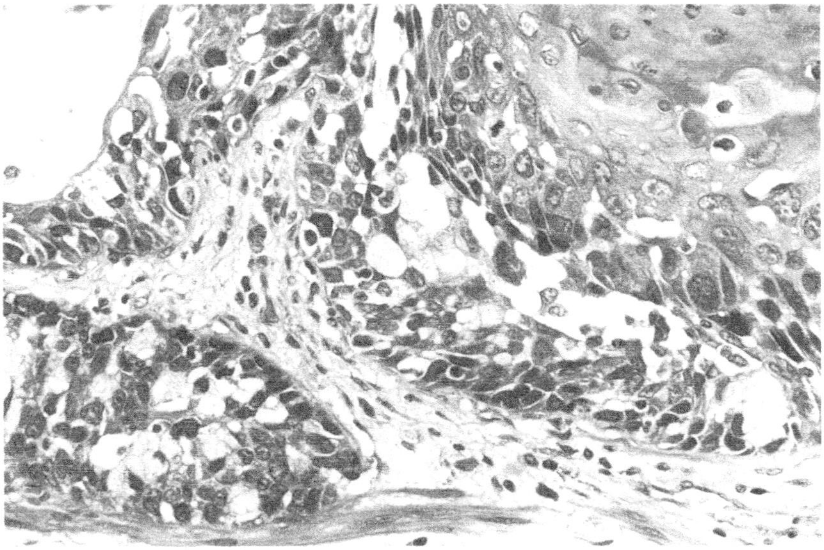

Fig. 17. *Mucoepidermoid carcinoma, oesophagus.* Same case as Fig. 16

×75

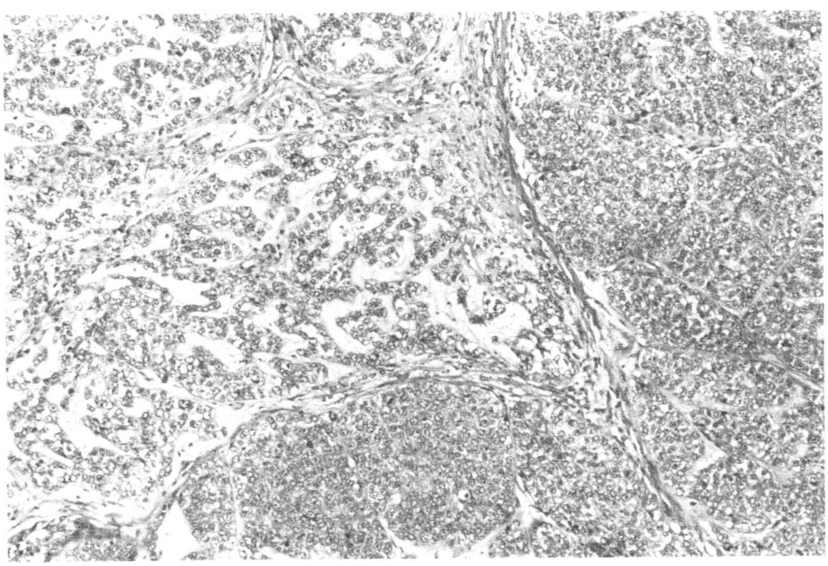

Fig. 18. *Adenoid cystic carcinoma, oesophagus*

× 150

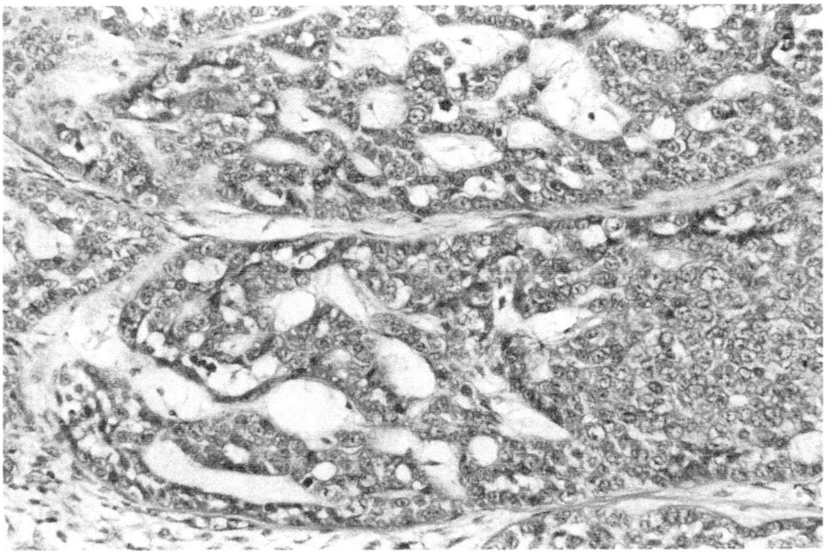

Fig. 19. *Adenoid cystic carcinoma, oesophagus.* Same case as Fig. 18

× 75

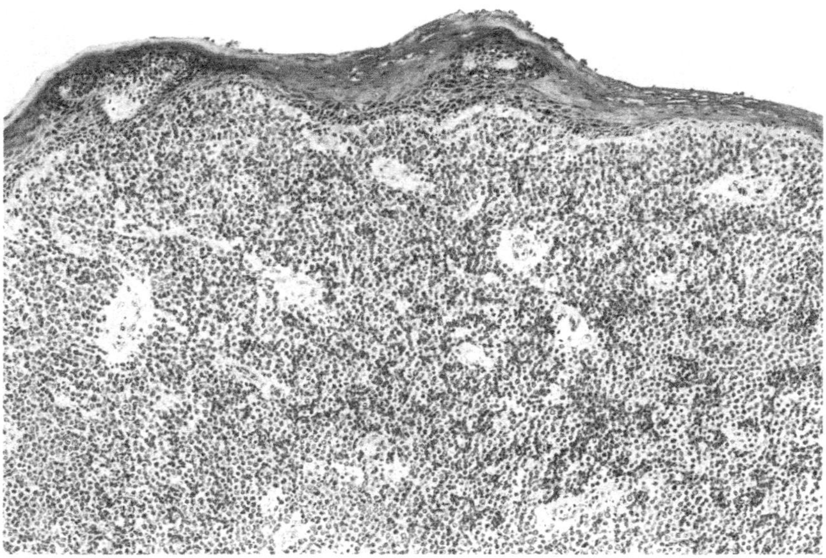

Fig. 20. *Small cell carcinoma, oesophagus*

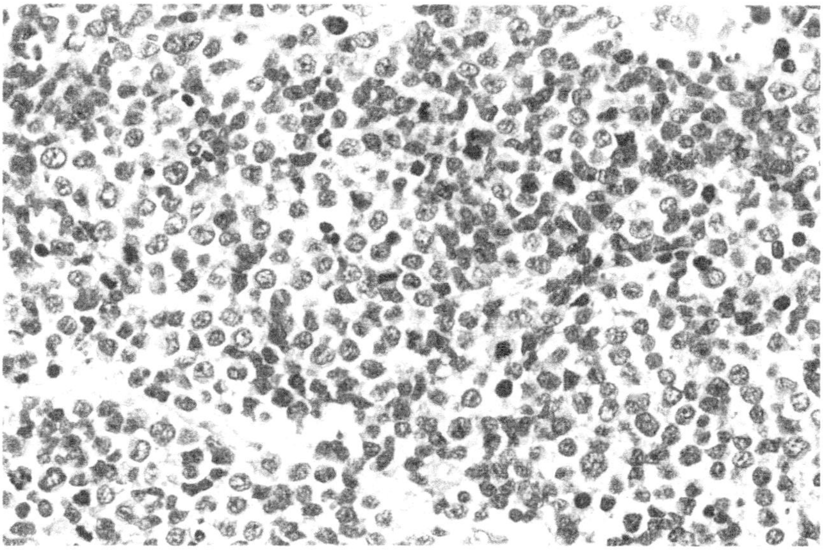

× 300

Fig. 21. *Small cell carcinoma, oesophagus.* Same case as Fig. 20. Round cells. Mitoses

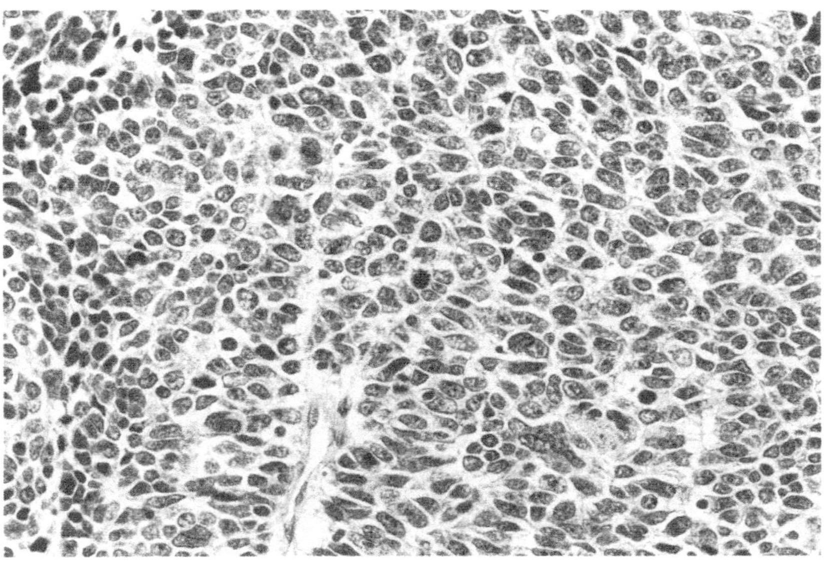

× 300

Fig. 22. *Small cell carcinoma, oesophagus.* Round to spindle cells

× 150

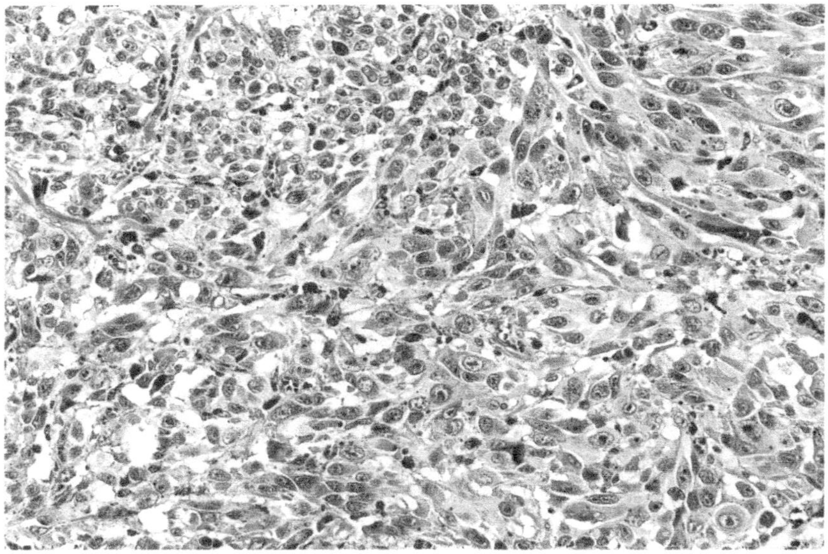

Fig. 23. *Malignant melanoma, oesophagus.* Melanin is seen
(Colour illustration see p. 105)

× 75

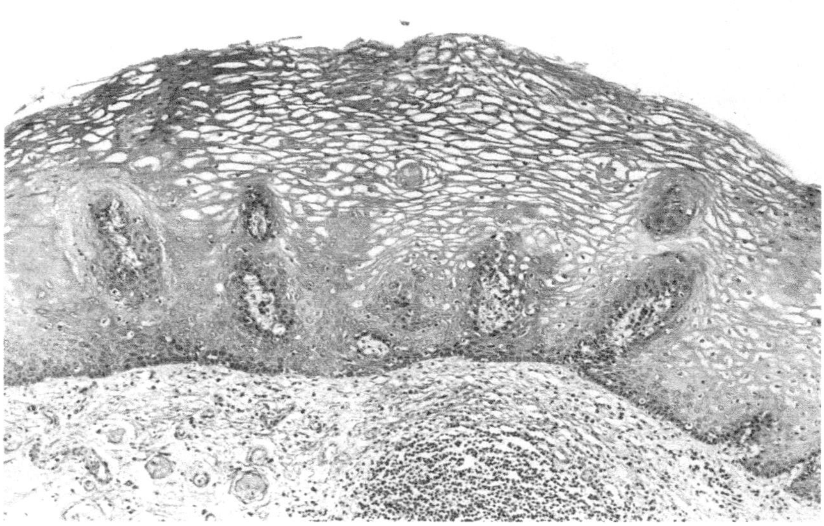

Fig. 24. *Glycogenic acanthosis, oesophagus*

× 30

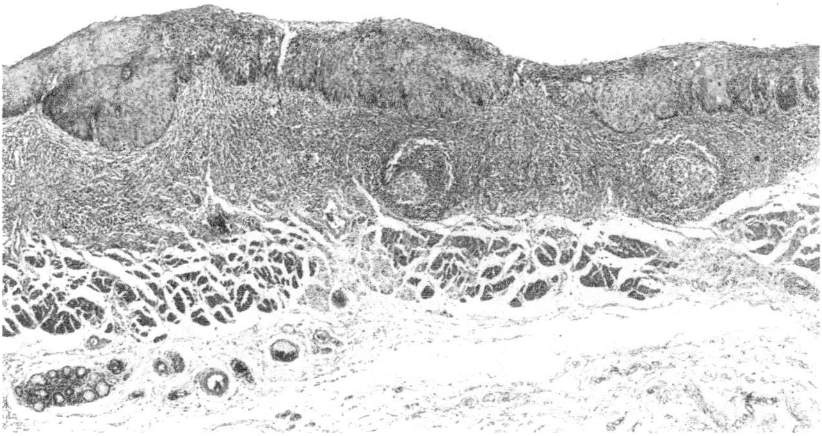

Fig. 25. *Carcinoma in situ, oesophagus.* Flat lesion measuring 33 × 10 mm

× 150

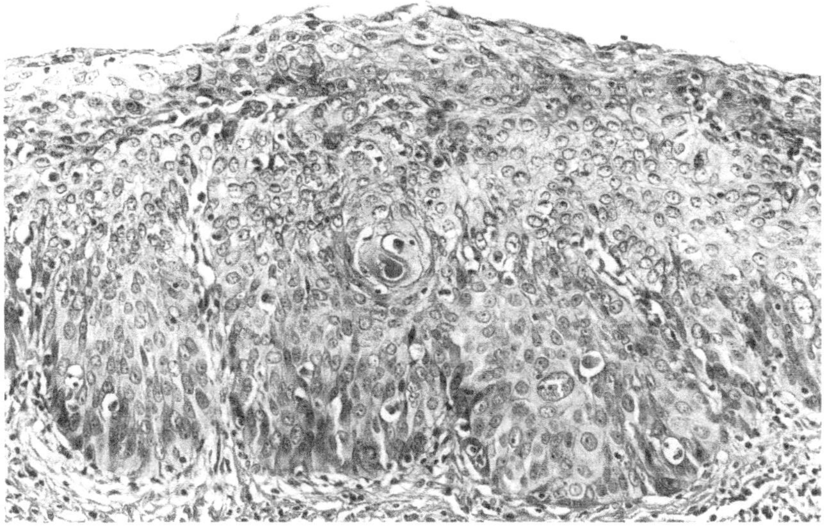

Fig. 26. *Carcinoma in situ, oesophagus.* Same case as Fig. 25

× 150

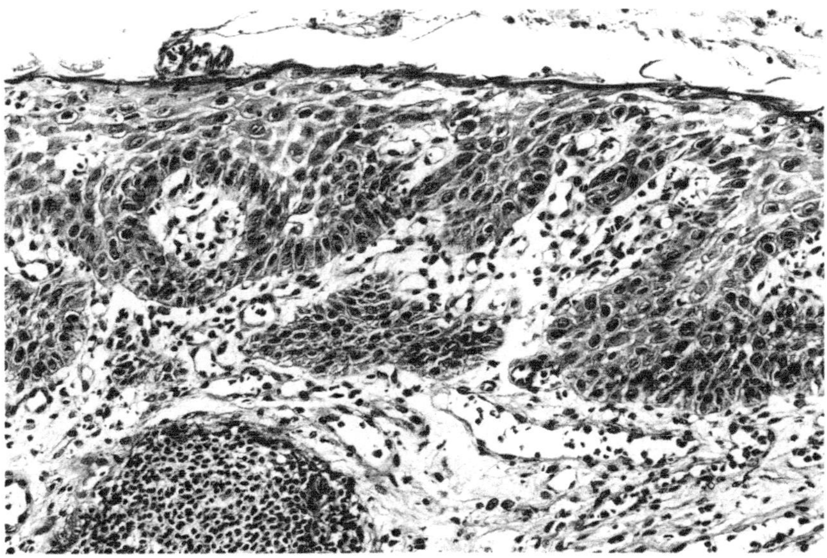

Fig. 27. *Reflux oesophagitis*. Immature regenerating epithelium in biopsy specimen

× 30

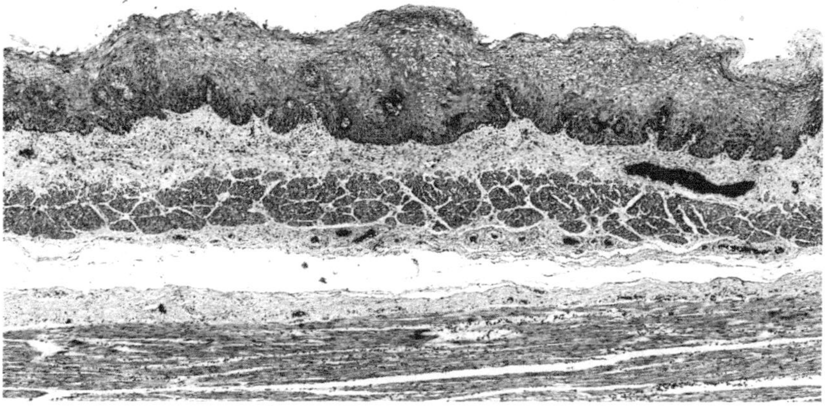

Fig. 28. *Chronic oesophagitis*. Focal lesion found in resected oesophagus with a squamous cell carcinoma invading submucosa

× 150

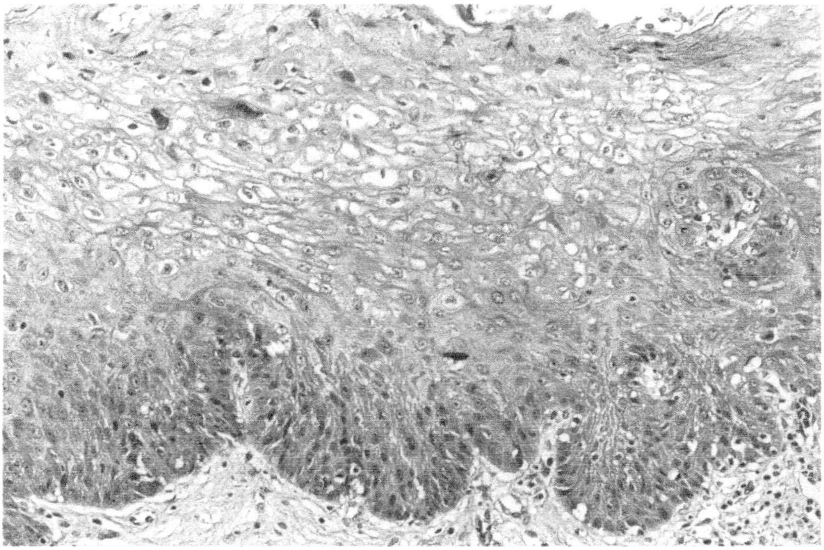

Fig. 29. *Chronic oesophagitis*. Orderly gradual epithelial maturation with well-preserved nuclear polarity, cell differentiation and distinct intercellular bridges. Same case as Fig. 28

× 30

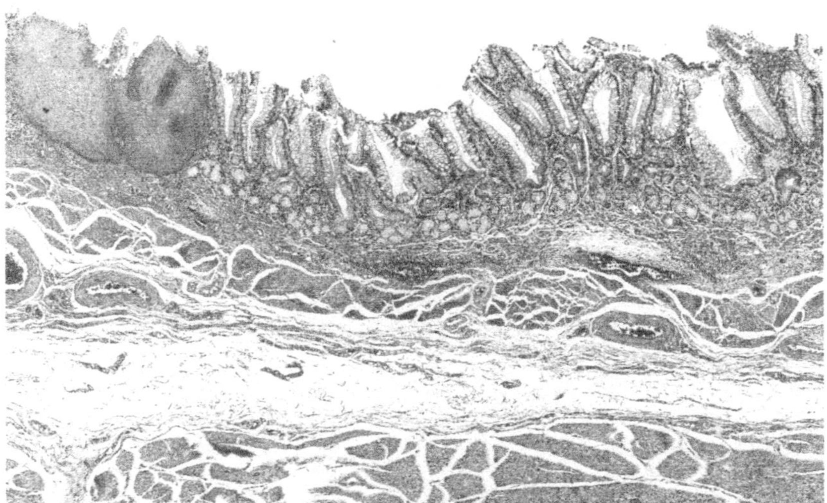

Fig. 30. *Barrett oesophagus*. Incomplete type intestinal metaplasia and pseudopyloric glands

×75

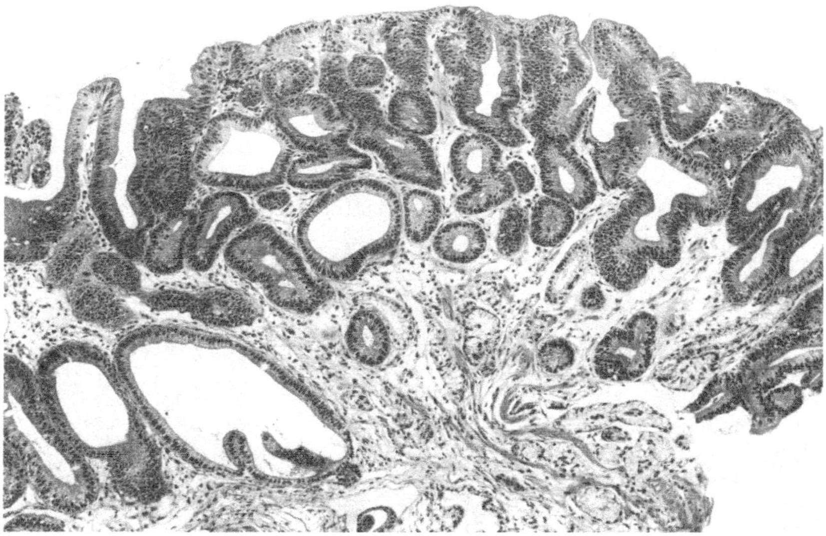

Fig. 31. *Tubular adenoma, stomach.* Biopsy specimen from small sessile polyp

×300

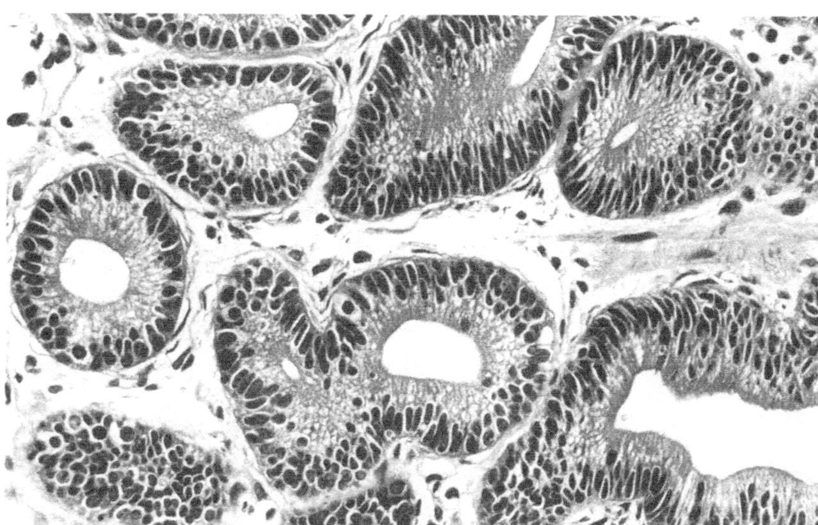

Fig. 32. *Tubular adenoma, stomach.* Same case as Fig. 31

× 30

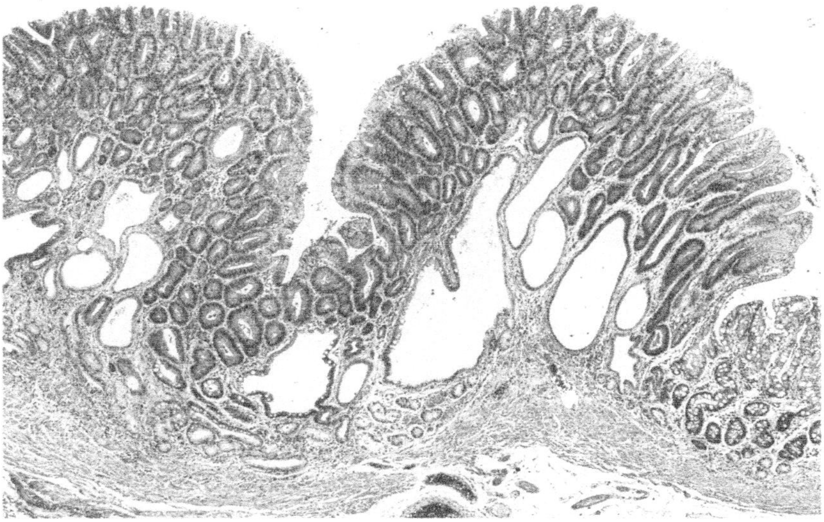

Fig. 33. *Tubular adenoma, stomach.* Sessile polypoid lesion measuring 10 × 8 mm

× 150

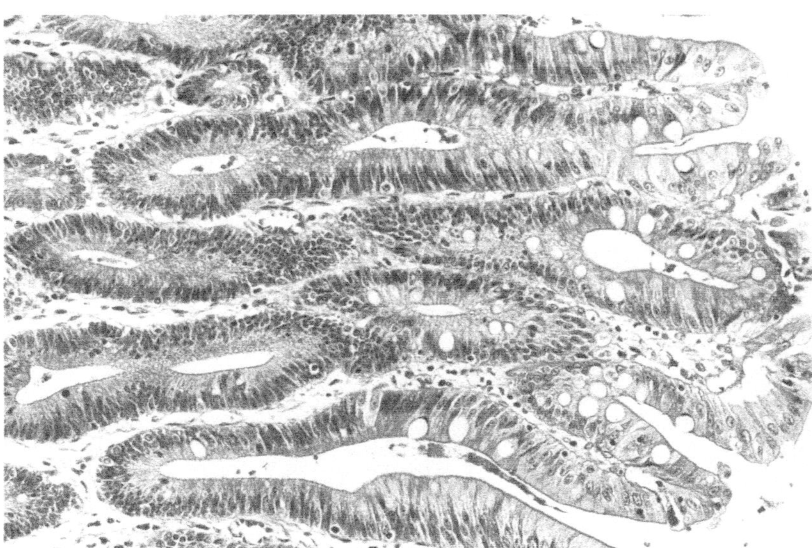

Fig. 34. *Tubular adenoma, stomach.* Same case as Fig. 33

× 30

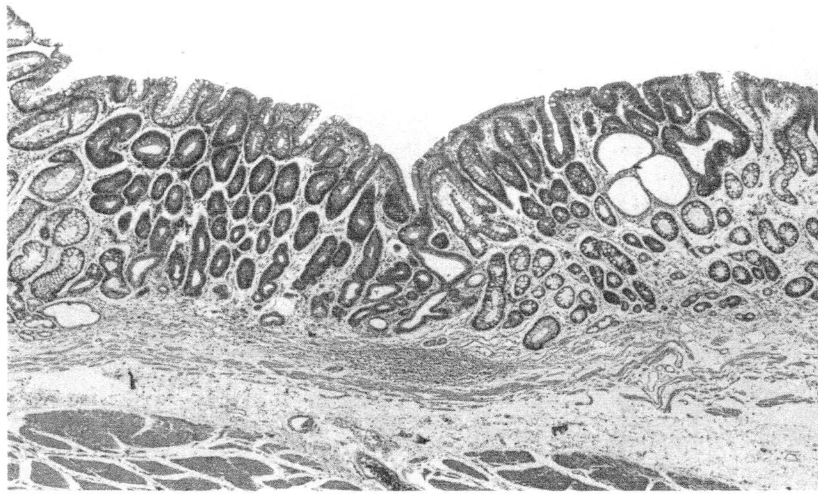

Fig. 35. *Tubular adenoma, stomach.* Depressed lesion measuring 2.7 × 2 mm (Colour illustration see p. 105)

× 300

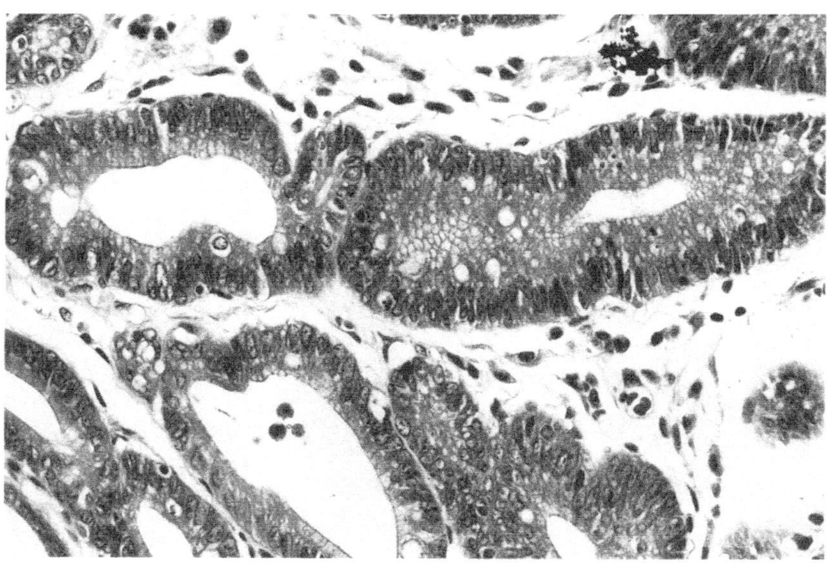

Fig. 36. *Tubular adenoma, stomach.* Same case as Fig. 35

×8

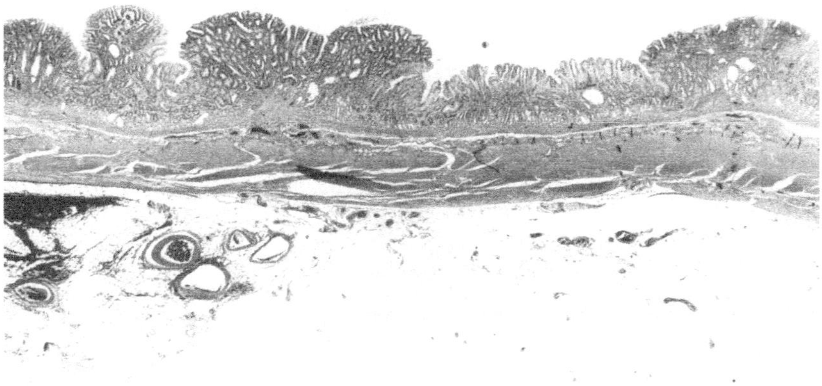

Fig. 37. *Tubular adenomas, stomach.* Over 70 adenomas, sessile polypoid, flat and depressed types, limited to gastric antral or intestinalized mucosa were in this patient with familial adenomatosis coli

×300

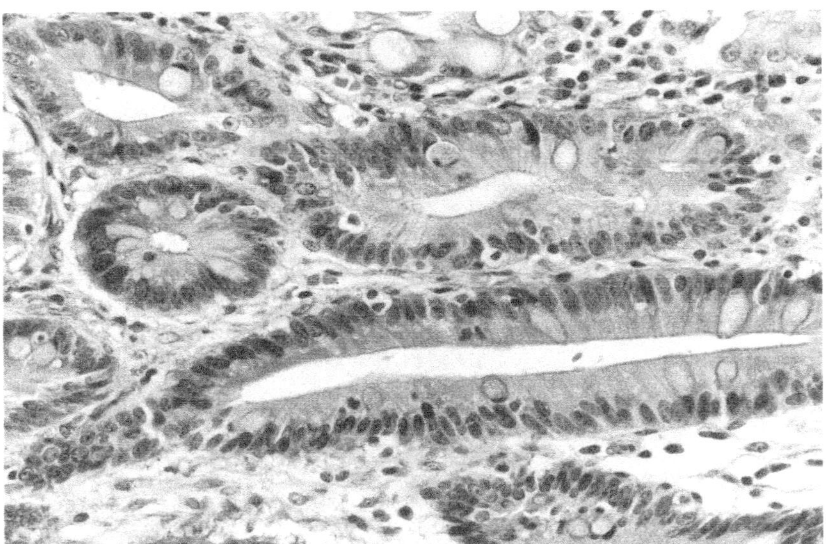

Fig. 38. *Tubular adenoma, stomach.* Same case as Fig. 37

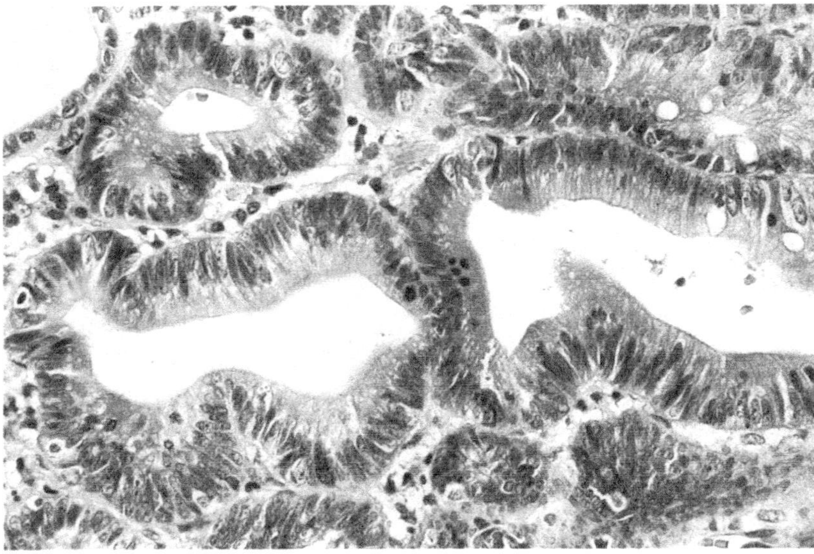

× 300

Fig. 39. *Tubular adenoma, stomach.* Magnification of the upper right part of Fig. 44

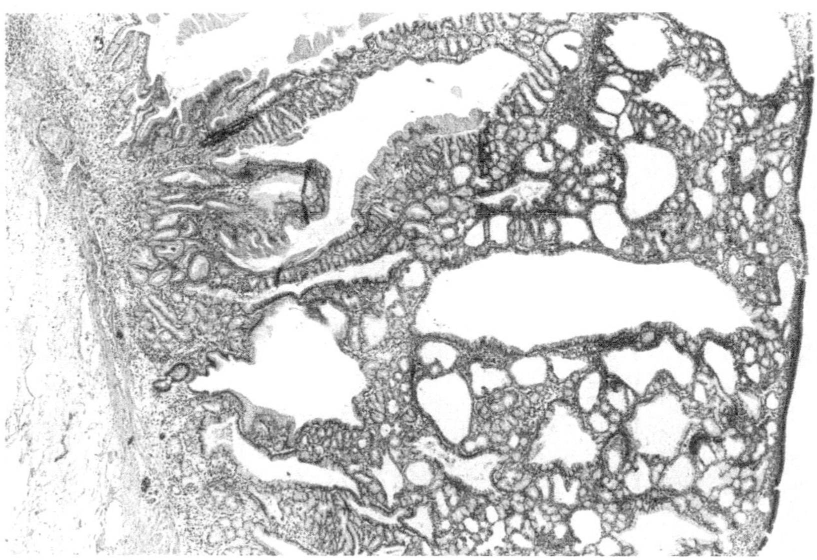

× 30

Fig. 40. *Tubular adenoma, stomach.* Polypoid pyloric gland-type lesion in gastric fornix

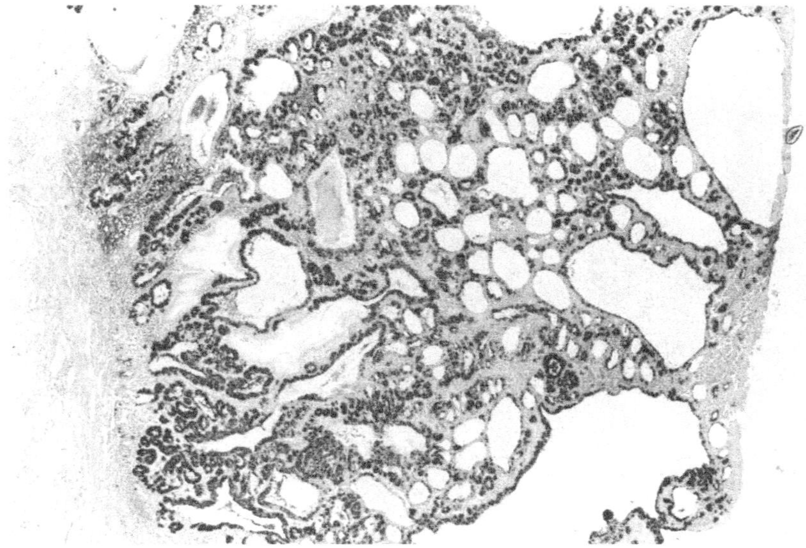

× 30

Fig. 41. *Tubular adenoma, stomach.* Intracellular mucin stained brown with paradoxical concanavalin A staining (pyloric gland-type mucin). Same case as Fig. 40

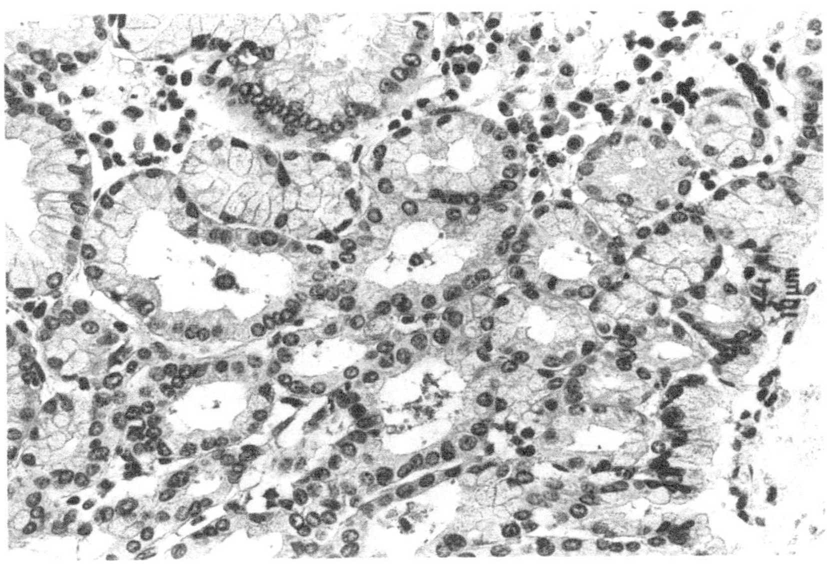

× 300

Fig. 42. *Tubular adenoma, stomach.* Pyloric gland-type adenoma with much mucin

×75

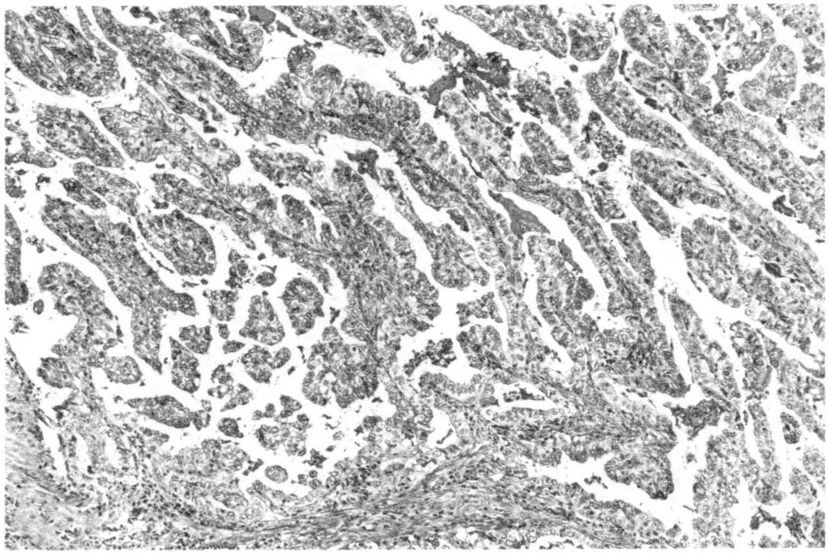

Fig. 43. *Papillary adenocarcinoma, stomach.* Submucosal part of advanced carcinoma

×30

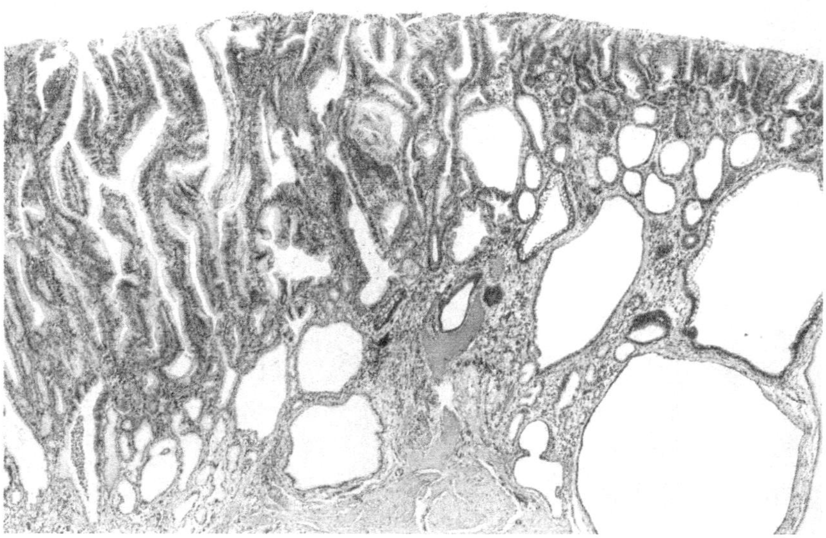

Fig. 44. *Papillotubular adenocarcinoma in adenoma, stomach.* Sessile polypoid lesion, 23 × 20 mm. Left, intramucosal carcinoma; right, adenoma. See Fig. 39

× 300

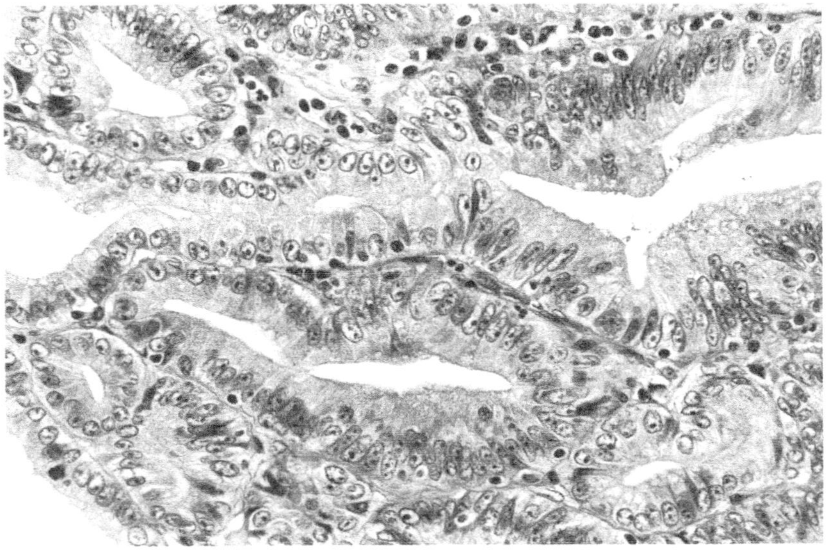

Fig. 45. *Papillotubular adenocarcinoma, stomach.* Magnification of tubular part in lower left part of Fig. 44

× 75

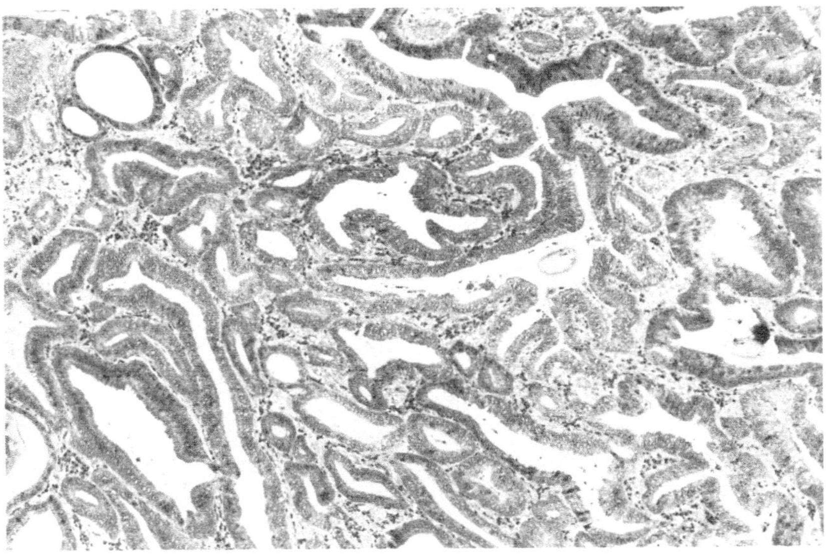

Fig. 46. *Papillotubular adenocarcinoma, stomach.* Sessile polypoid lesion, 11 × 8 mm, of intramucosal carcinoma

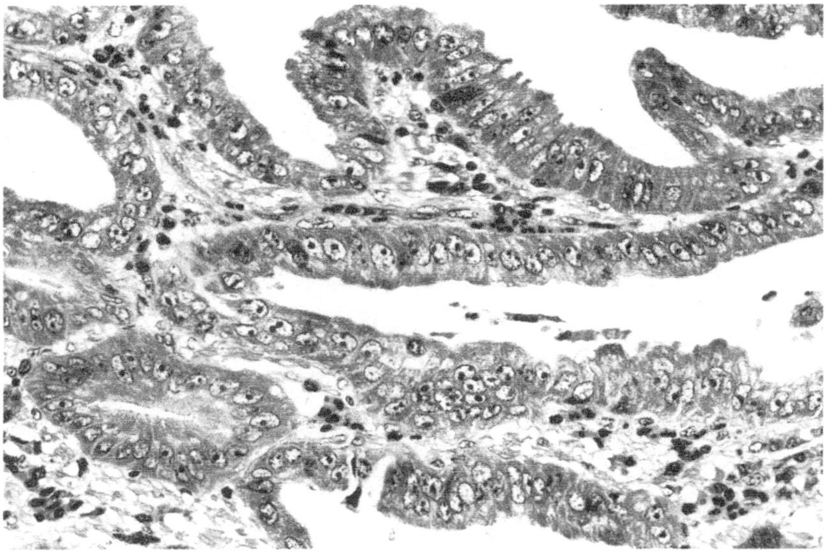

× 300

Fig. 47. *Papillotubular adenocarcinoma, stomach*. Enlarged, round or oval, vesicular nuclei with dotted chromatin and enlarged distinct eosinophilic nucleoli. Magnification of central part of Fig. 46

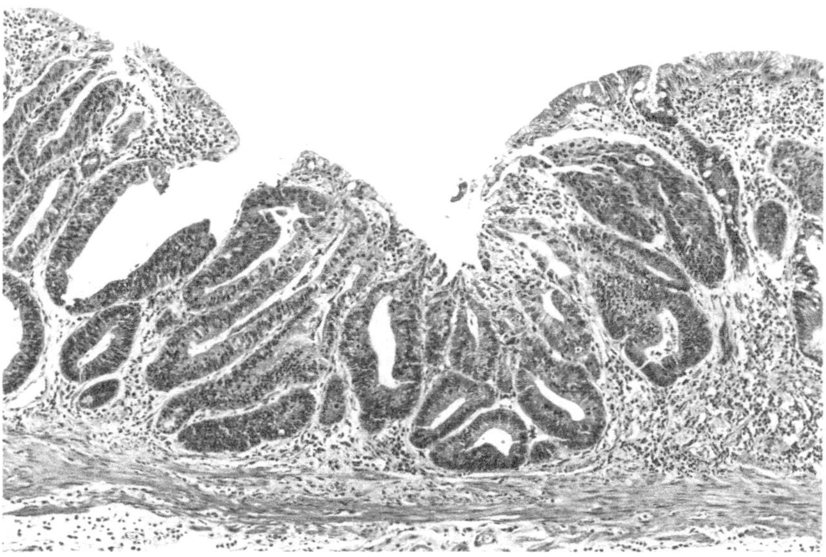

× 75

Fig. 48. *Tubular adenocarcinoma, stomach*. Well differentiated. Mucosal part of depressed type carcinoma, 8 × 6 mm, which invaded submucosa

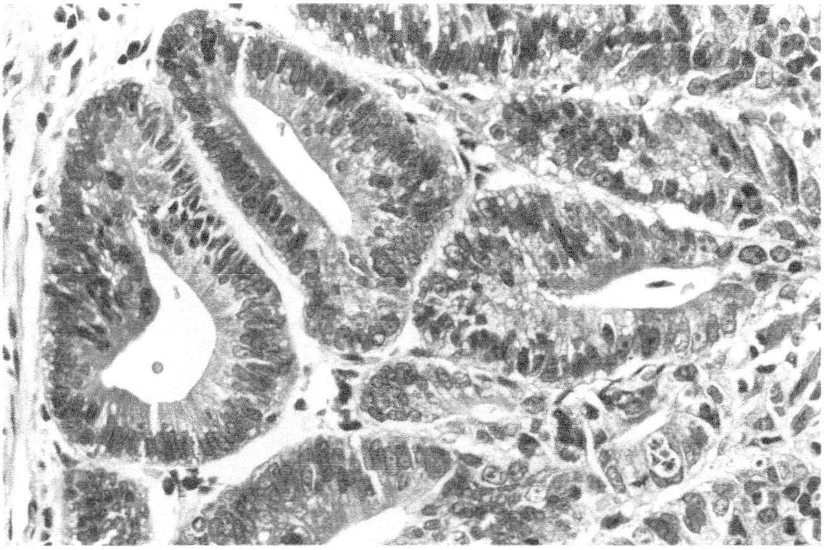

× 300

Fig. 49. *Tubular adenocarcinoma, stomach.* Well differentiated. Magnification of central part of Fig. 48

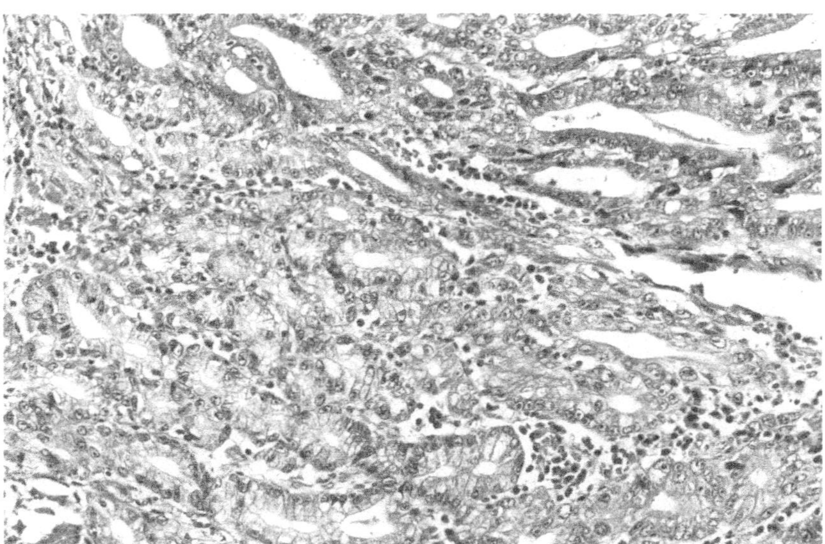

× 150

Fig. 50. *Tubular adenocarcinoma, stomach.* Well differentiated. Mucosal part of depressed-type carcinoma invading down to submucosa. Tumour cells have clear cytoplasm reminiscent of pyloric gland epithelium

× 30

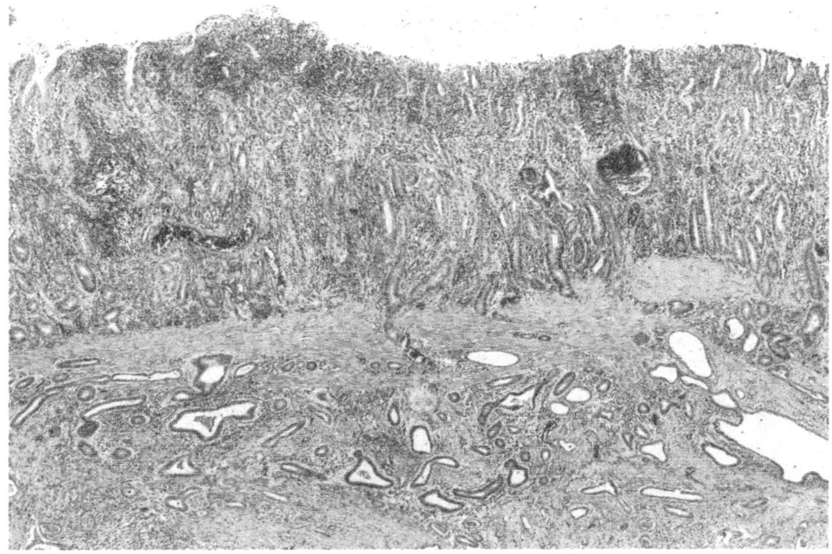

Fig. 51. *Tubular adenocarcinoma, stomach.* Well differentiated. Plateau-like polypoid lesion, 55 × 50 mm, extending into submucosa

× 300

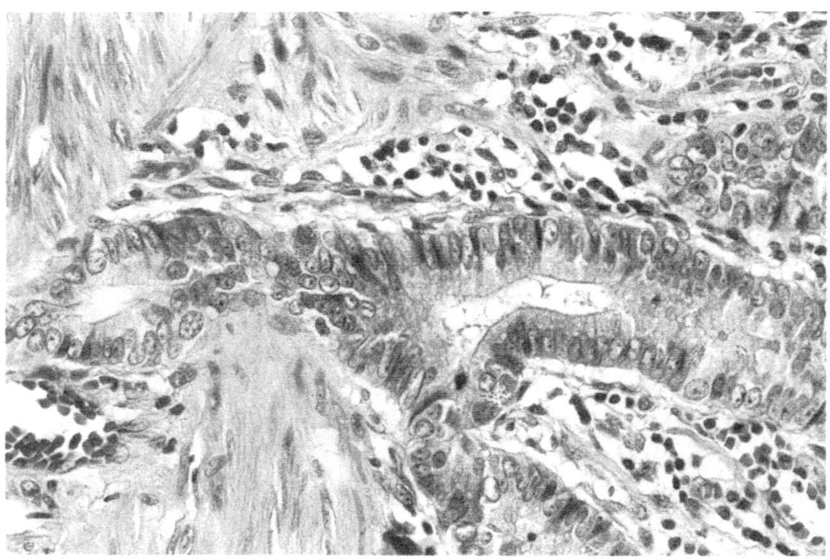

Fig. 52. *Tubular adenocarcinoma, stomach.* Well differentiated. Magnification of central part of Fig. 51. Tumour shows low-grade atypia and Paneth cell differentiation

×75

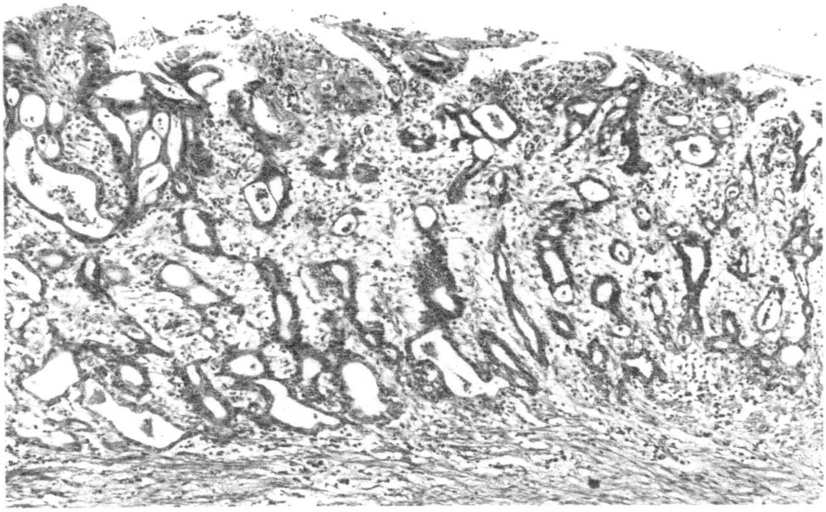

Fig. 53. *Tubular adenocarcinoma, stomach.* Moderately differentiated. Intramucosal carcinoma, depressed type, 48 × 28 mm

×75

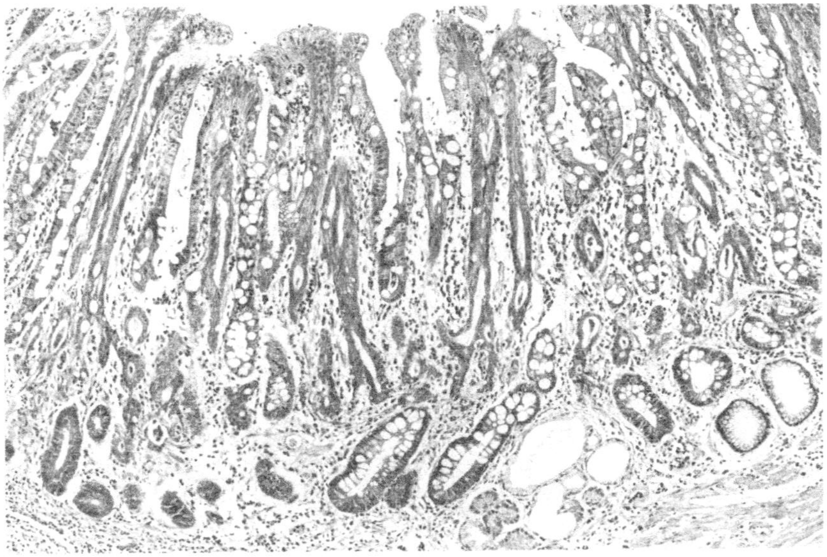

Fig. 54. *Tubular adenocarcinoma, stomach.* Moderately differentiated. Flat lesion of intramucosal carcinoma, 28 × 22 mm, with irregular branching and anastomosis of neoplastic tubules; non-neoplastic glands between and under them

× 300

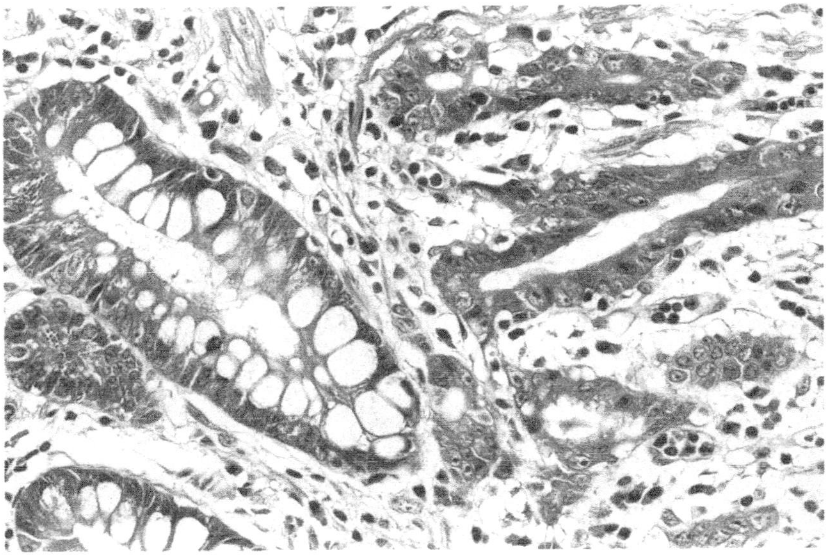

Fig. 55. *Tubular adenocarcinoma, stomach.* Moderately differentiated. Non-neoplastic glands of complete-type intestinal metaplasia are present under carcinoma. Same case as Fig. 54

× 150

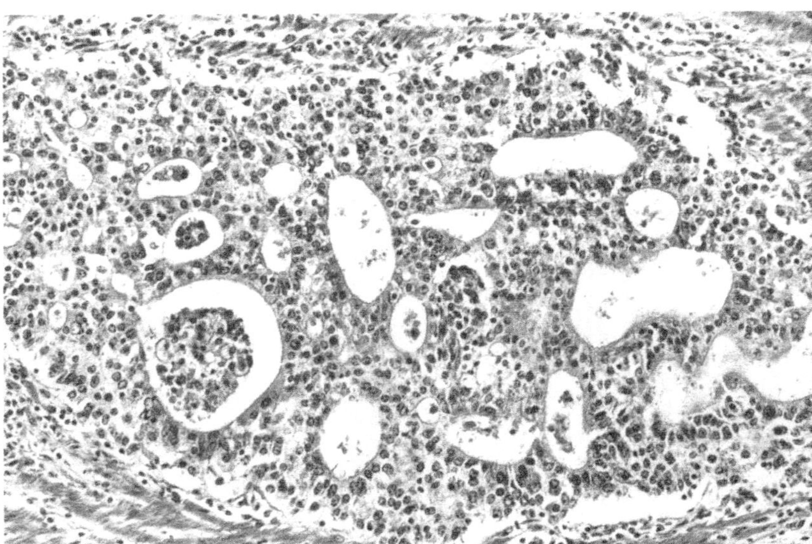

Fig. 56. *Tubular adenocarcinoma, stomach.* Moderately differentiated. Cribriform pattern. Advanced carcinoma in muscle

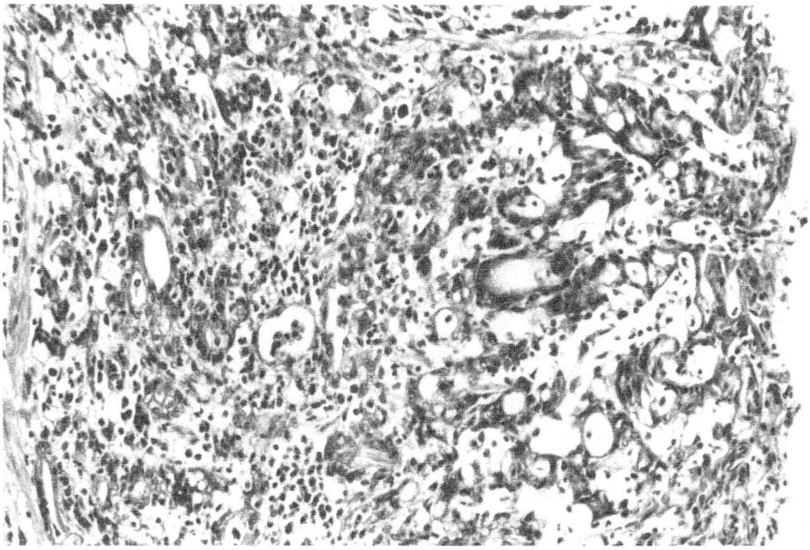

× 150

Fig. 57. *Tubular adenocarcinoma, stomach.* Poorly differentiated. Mucosal part of carcinoma which invaded submucosa

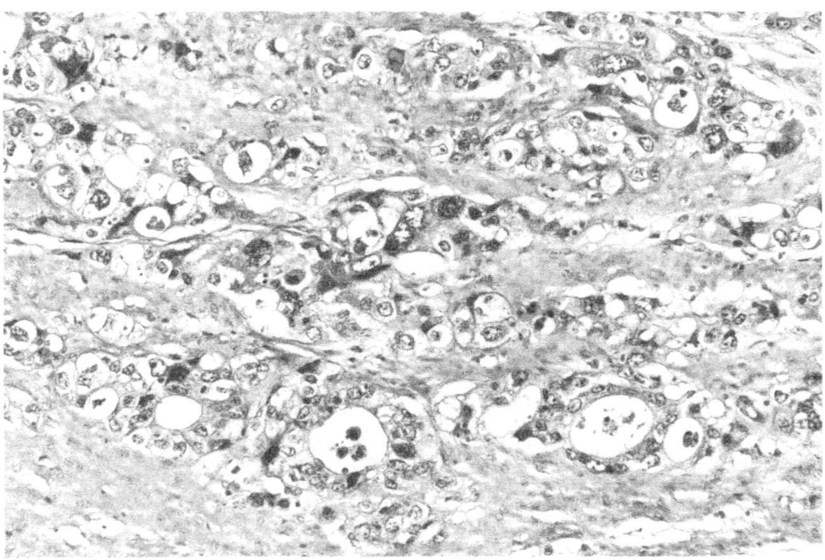

× 150

Fig. 58. *Tubular adenocarcinoma, stomach.* Poorly differentiated. Advanced carcinoma in muscle

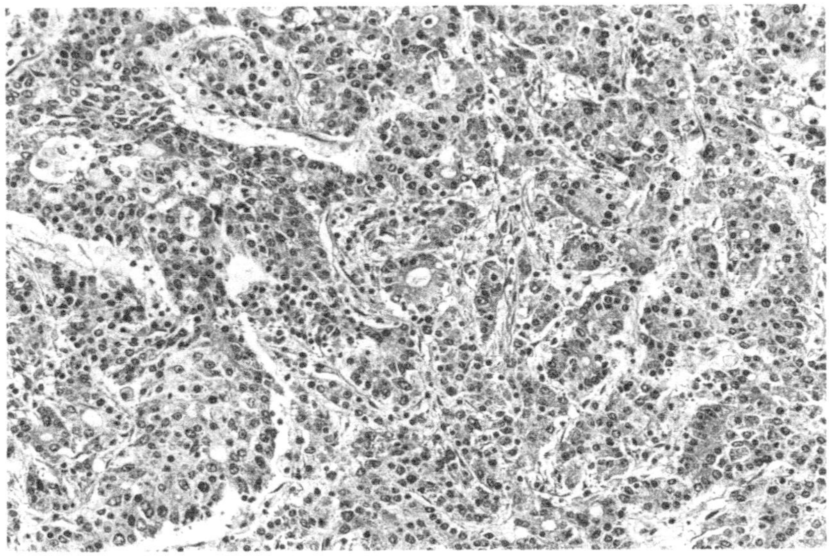

× 150

Fig. 59. *Tubular adenocarcinoma, stomach.* Poorly differentiated. Solid structure with acini. Subserosal part

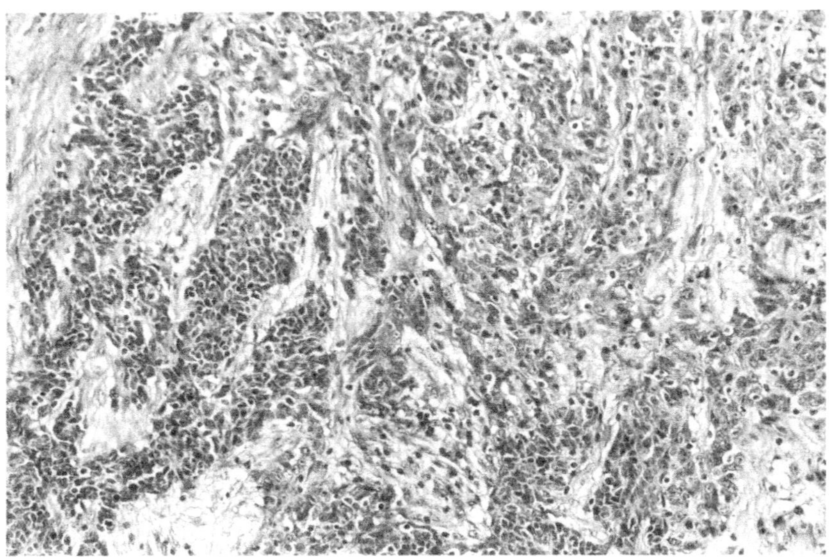

× 150

Fig. 60. *Tubular adenocarcinoma, stomach.* Poorly differentiated. Solid structure. Grimelius stain was negative

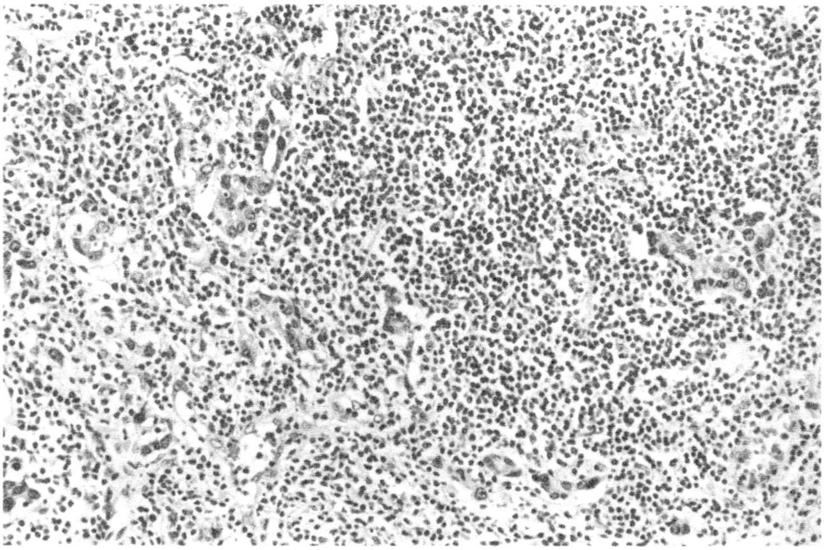

× 150

Fig. 61. *Tubular adenocarcinoma, stomach.* Poorly differentiated. Lymphoid stroma
(Colour illustration see p. 106)

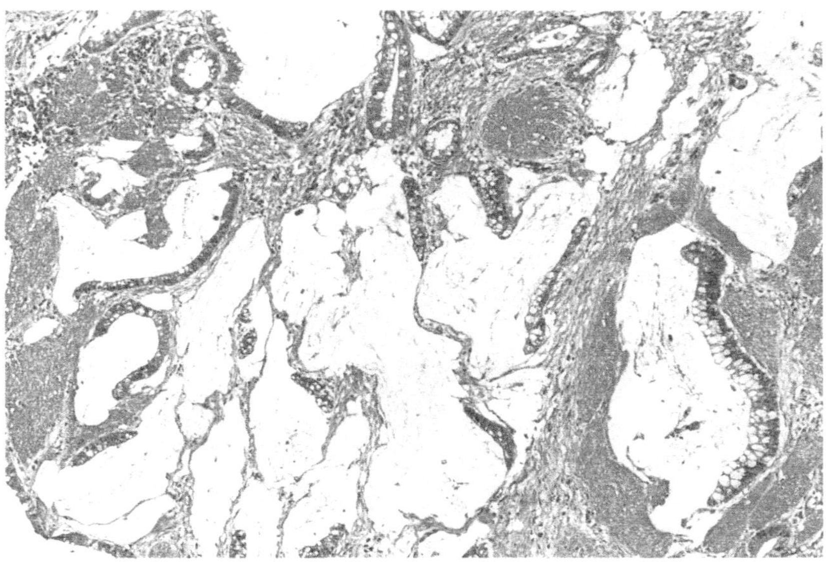

× 75

Fig. 62. *Mucinous adenocarcinoma, stomach.* Well differentiated

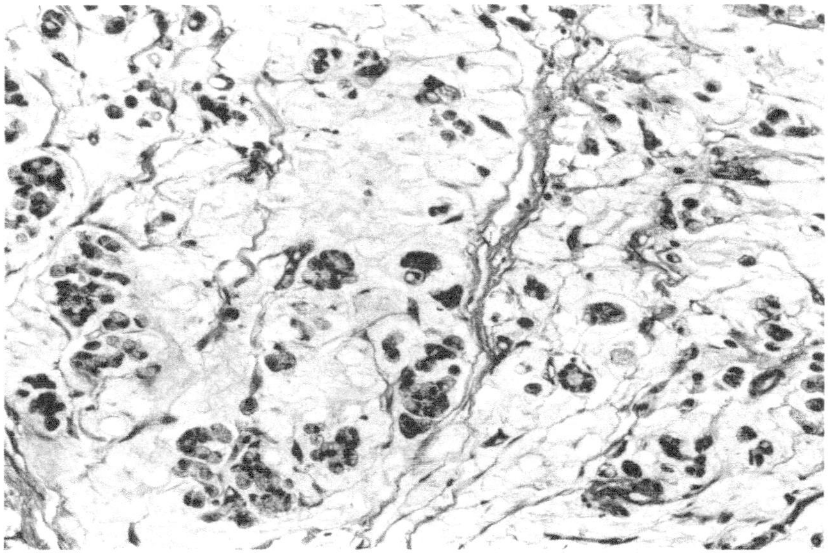

× 150

Fig. 63. *Mucinous adenocarcinoma, stomach.* Poorly differentiated

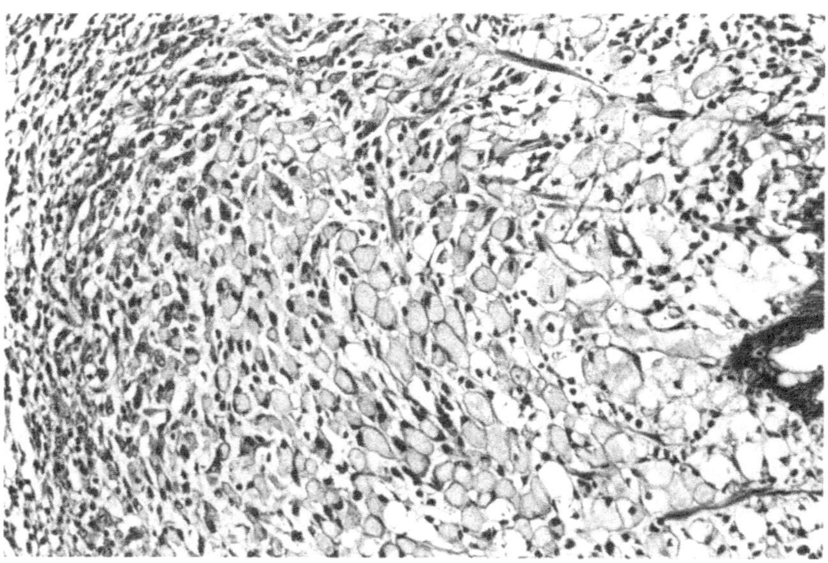

× 150

Fig. 64. *Signet-ring cell carcinoma, stomach.*
Two-layered pattern in intramucosal carcinoma, 12 × 9 mm
(Colour illustration see p. 106)

× 150

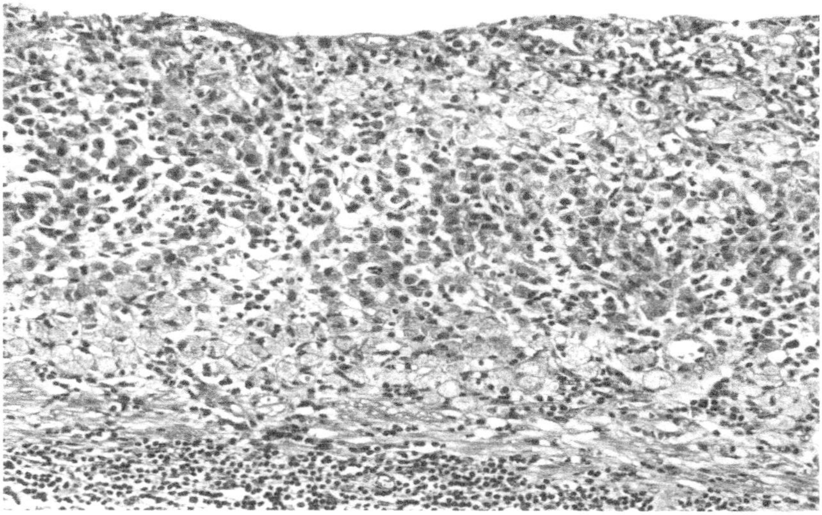

Fig. 65. *Signet-ring cell carcinoma, stomach.* Three-layered pattern with mucus containing cells in upper and lower layers. Mucosal part of advanced carcinoma

× 300

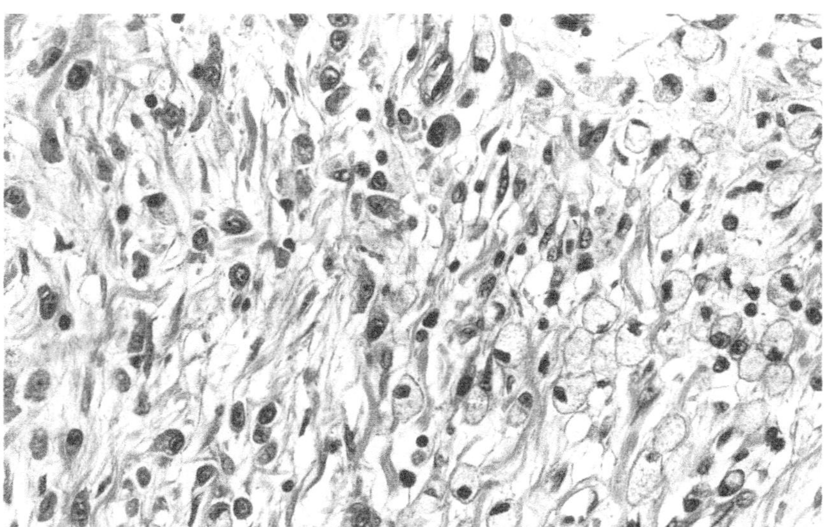

Fig. 66. *Signet-ring cell carcinoma, stomach.* Cells with or without mucin. Scirrhous growth pattern in submucosal part of advanced carcinoma

× 150

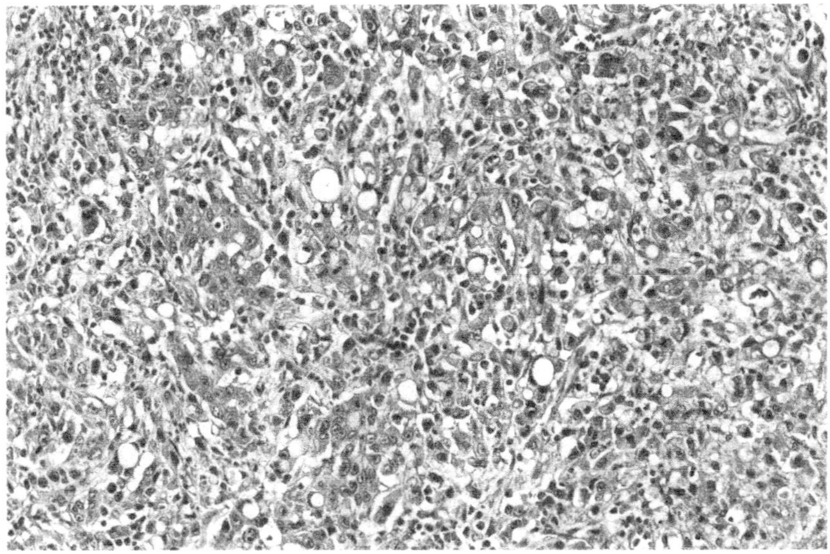

Fig. 67. *Signet-ring cell carcinoma, stomach.* Mucosal part of advanced carcinoma

× 300

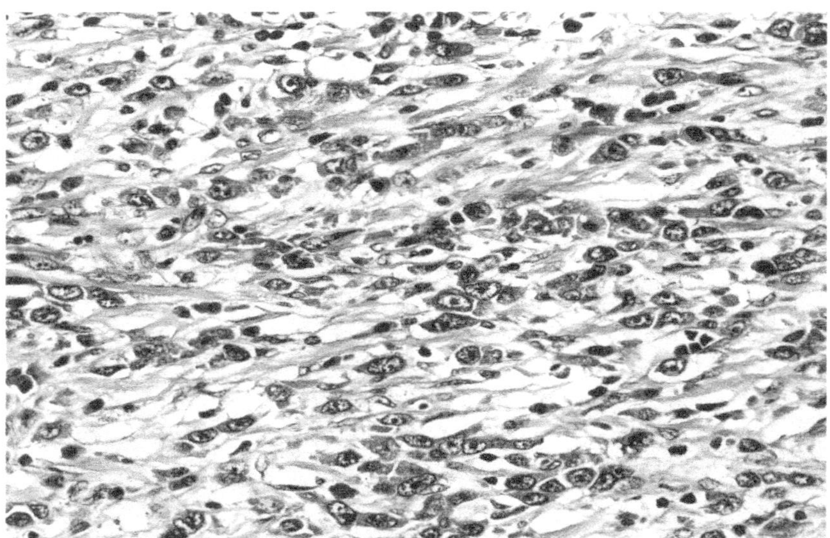

Fig. 68. *Signet-ring cell carcinoma, stomach.* Tumour cells have no mucin in this submucosal area. Same case as Fig. 67

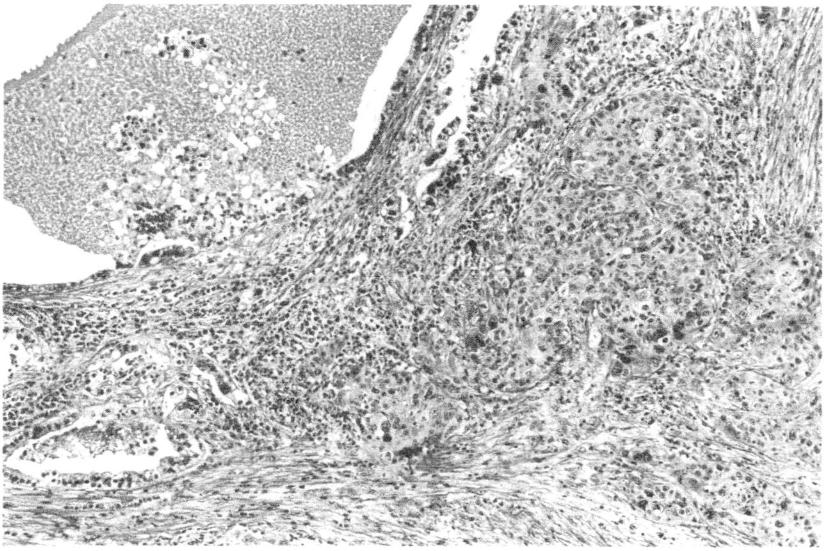

×75

Fig. 69. *Adenosquamous carcinoma, stomach.* Tumour located in gastric antrum

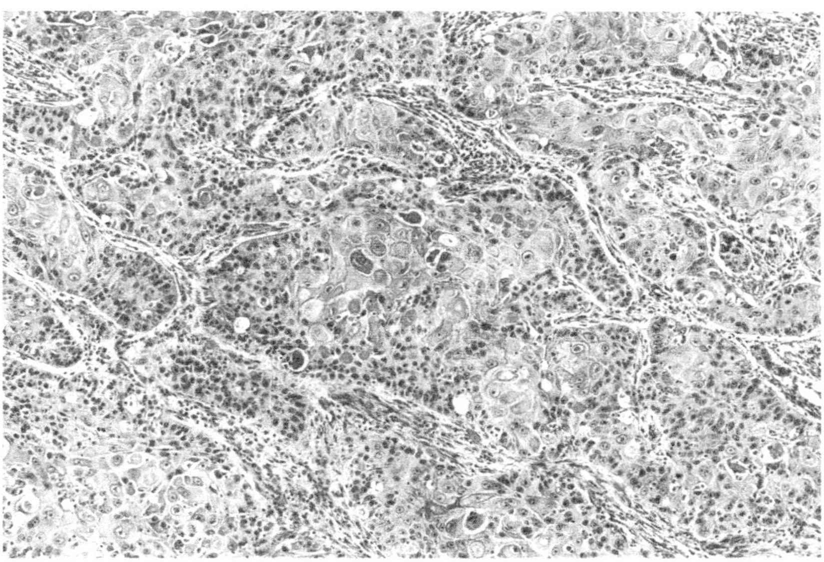

×75

Fig. 70. *Squamous cell carcinoma, stomach.* Tumour located in gastric body

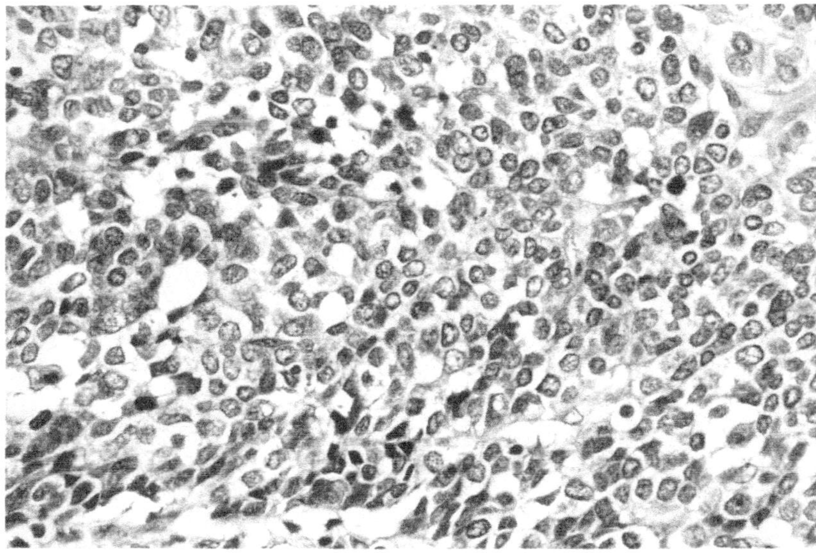

×300

Fig. 71. *Small cell carcinoma, stomach.* Round and oval nuclei with finely distributed chromatin and inconspicuous nucleoli

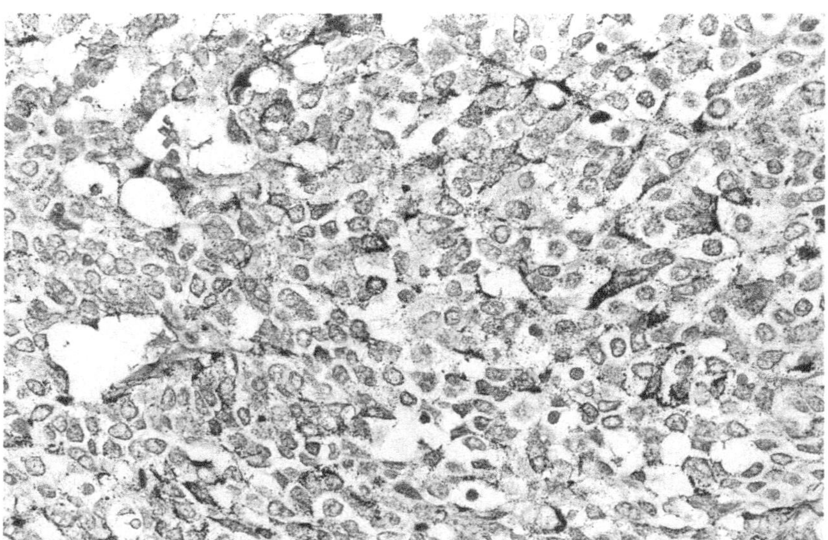

×300

Fig. 72. *Small cell carcinoma, stomach.* Grimelius staining demonstrates many black argyrophil granules in every cell. Same case as Fig. 71

× 75

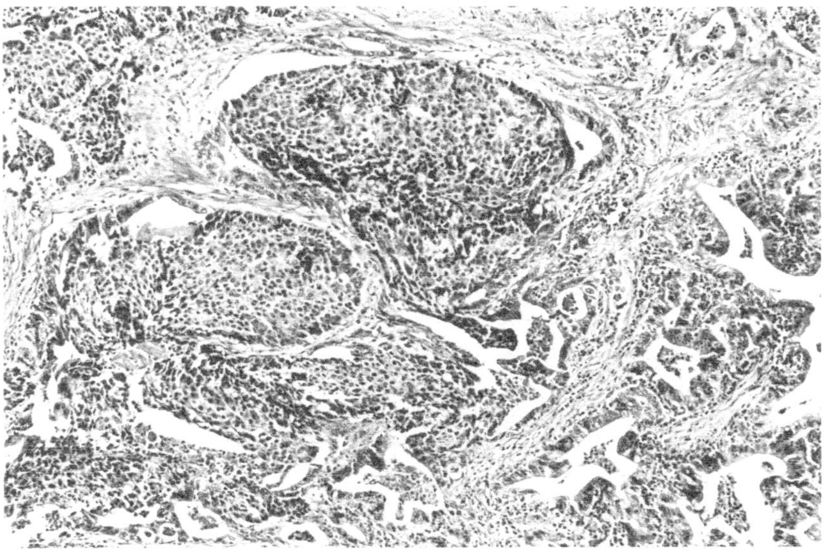

Fig. 73. *Small cell carcinoma with adenocarcinoma, stomach.* Adenocarcinoma (*right;* luminal side) and small cell carcinoma are mixed

× 300

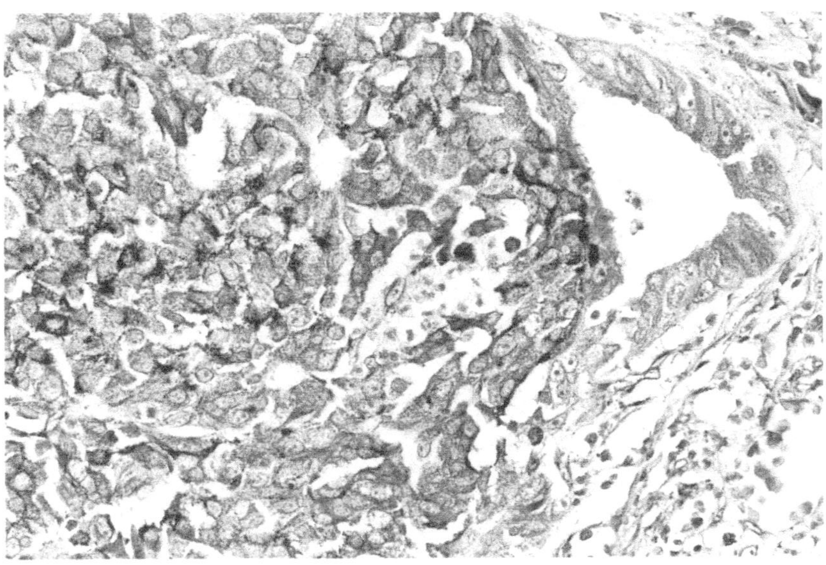

Fig. 74. *Small cell carcinoma with adenocarcinoma, stomach.* Grimelius staining for argyrophil granules is positive in small cell carcinoma, but negative in adenocarcinoma. Same case as Fig. 73

×30

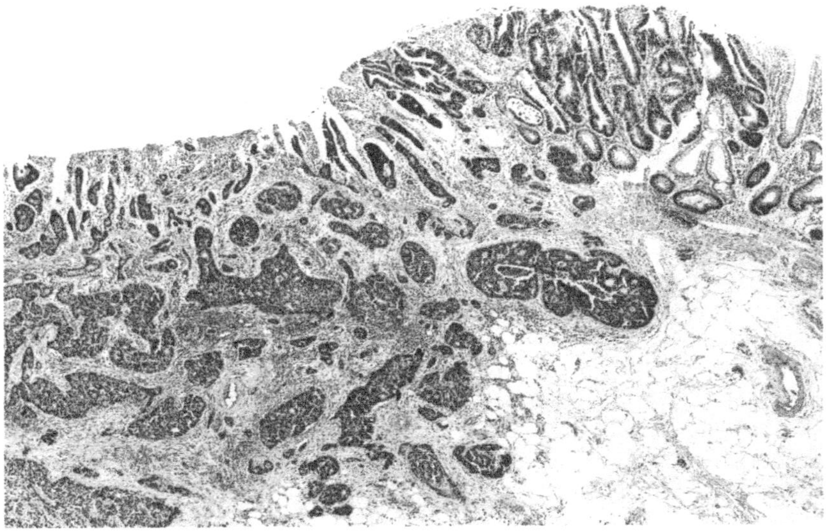

Fig. 75. *Small cell carcinoma with adenocarcinoma, stomach.* Tumour cells (argyrophil positive) invade into submucosa and show venous permeation. Liver metastasis found after 5 years

×300

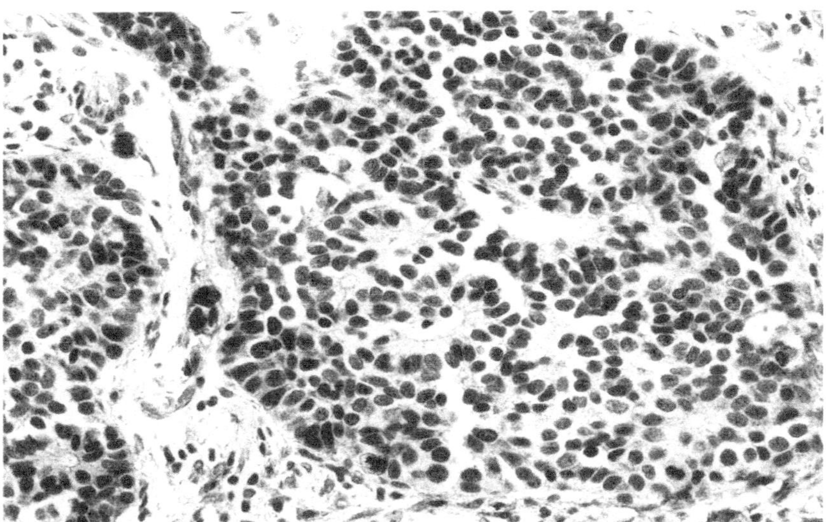

Fig. 76. *Small cell carcinoma, stomach.* Solid pattern with acini. Same case as Fig. 75

× 150

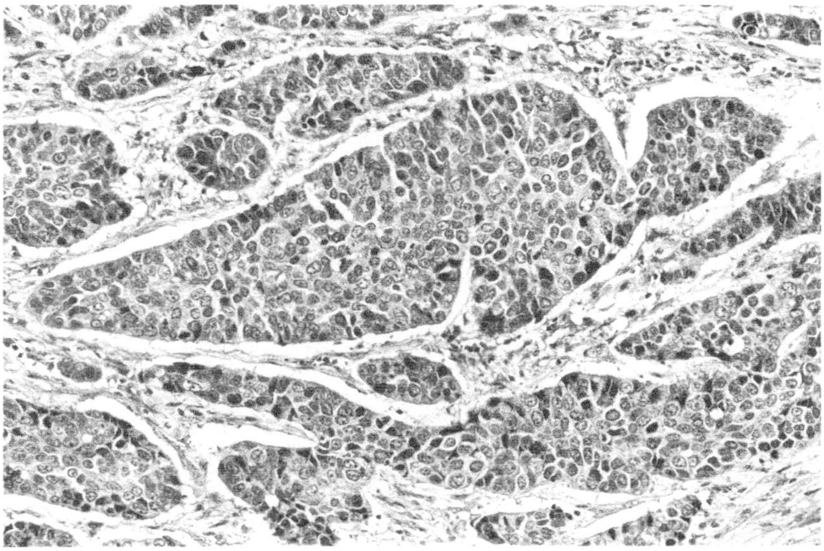

Fig. 77. *Undifferentiated carcinoma, stomach.* No argyrophil granules or mucin

× 75

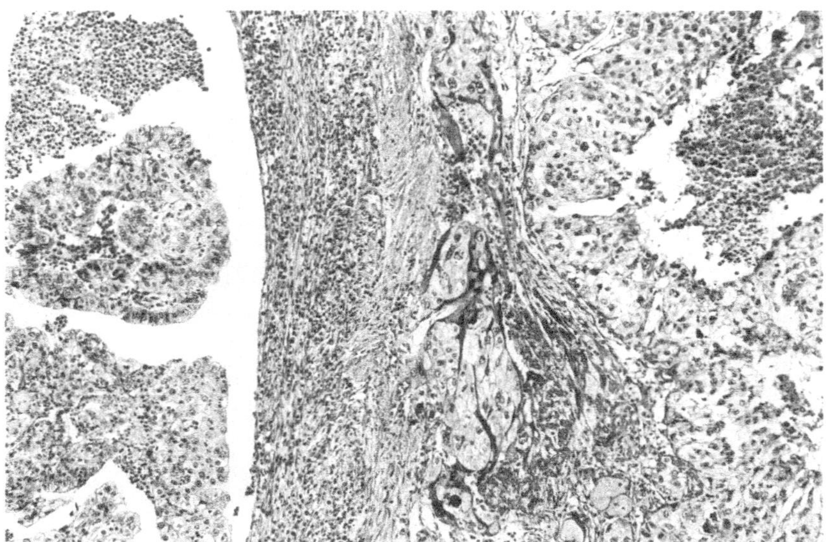

Fig. 78. *Choriocarcinoma, stomach.* Adenocarcinoma in left portion. A 53-year-old woman with high levels of human chorionic gonadotropin. No tumours in other organs

×75

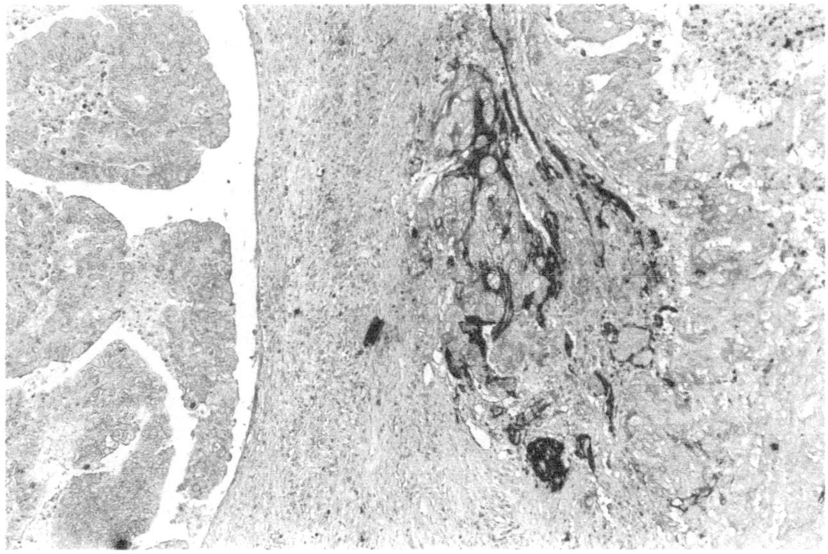

Fig. 79. *Choriocarcinoma, stomach.* Immunostaining of human chorionic gonadotrophin is positive in syncytiotrophoblasts. Same case as Fig. 78

×300

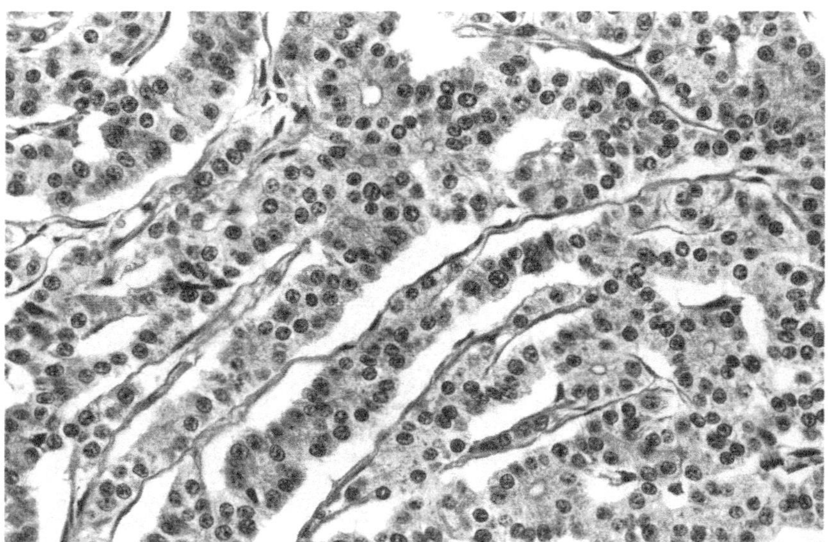

Fig. 80. *Carcinoid tumour, stomach.* Anastomosing trabecular structure with rosettes

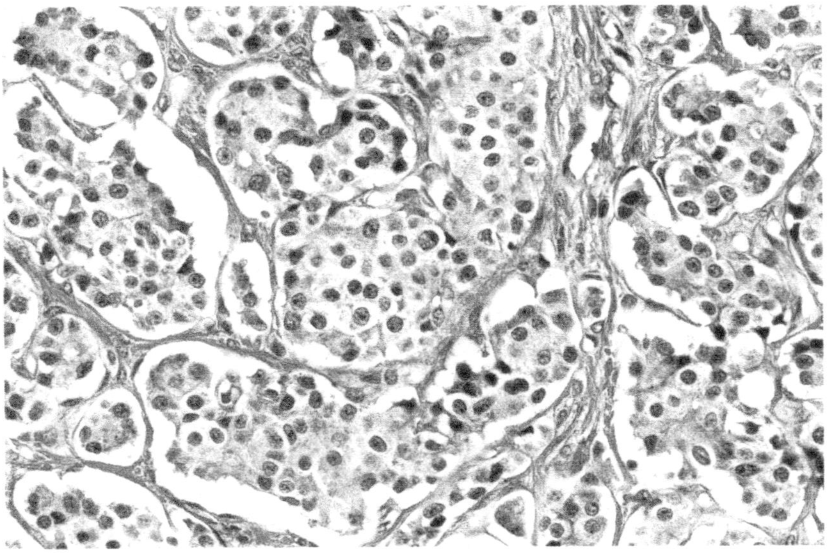

×300

Fig. 81. *Carcinoid tumour, stomach.* Small solid structure with rosette formation

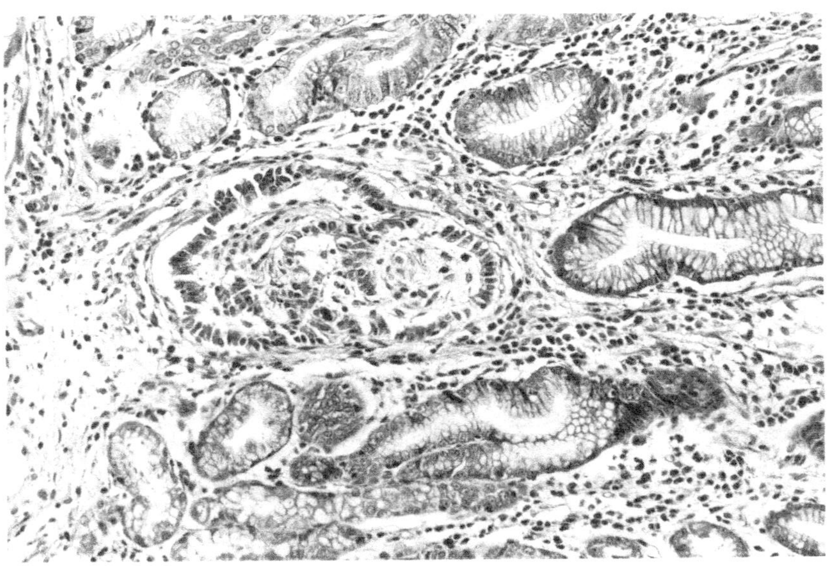

×75

Fig. 82. *Carcinoid tumour, stomach.* Microcarcinoid, 0.3 mm in largest diameter, in patient with type A gastritis

× 300

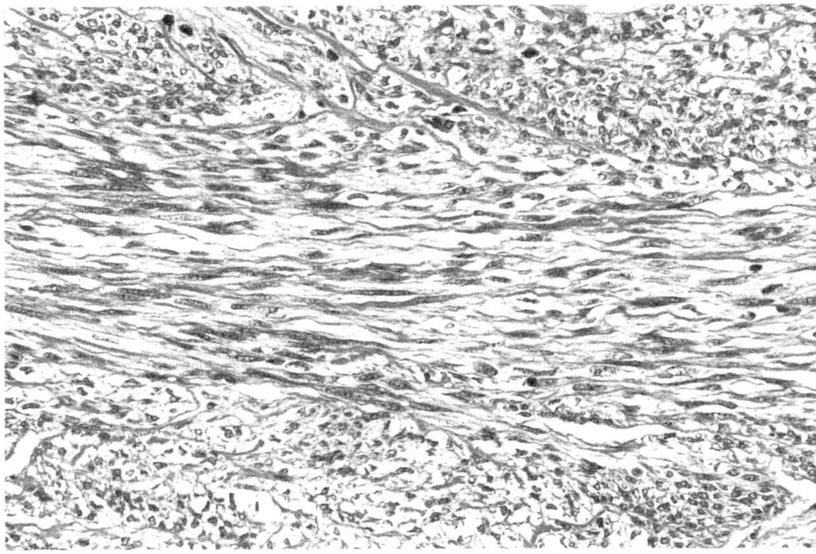

Fig. 83. *Leiomyoma, stomach*

× 300

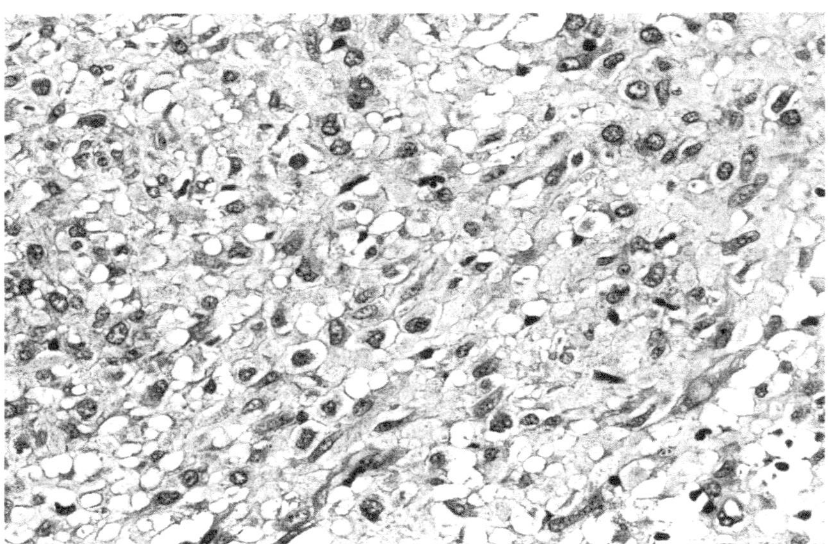

Fig. 84. *Epithelioid leiomyoma, stomach*

× 75

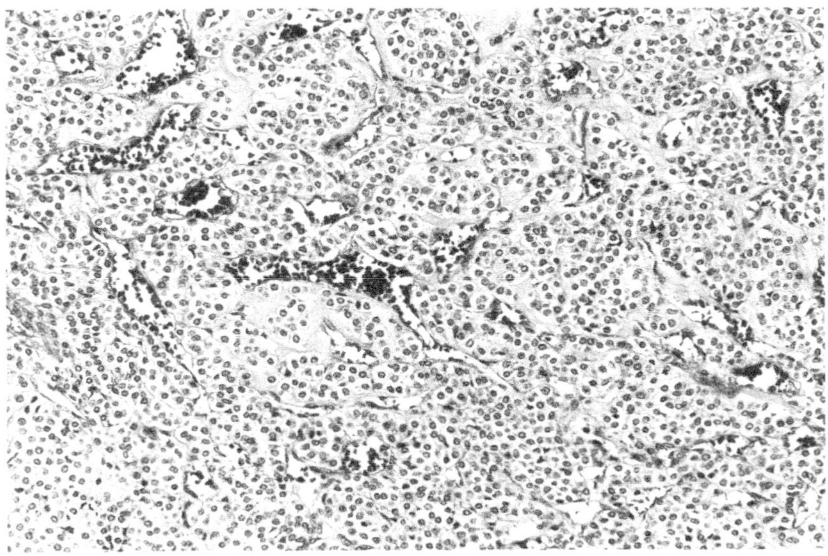

Fig. 85. *Glomus tumour, stomach.* Vascular tumour composed of acidophilic, epithelioid, round cells of uniform size with round and oval nuclei

× 75

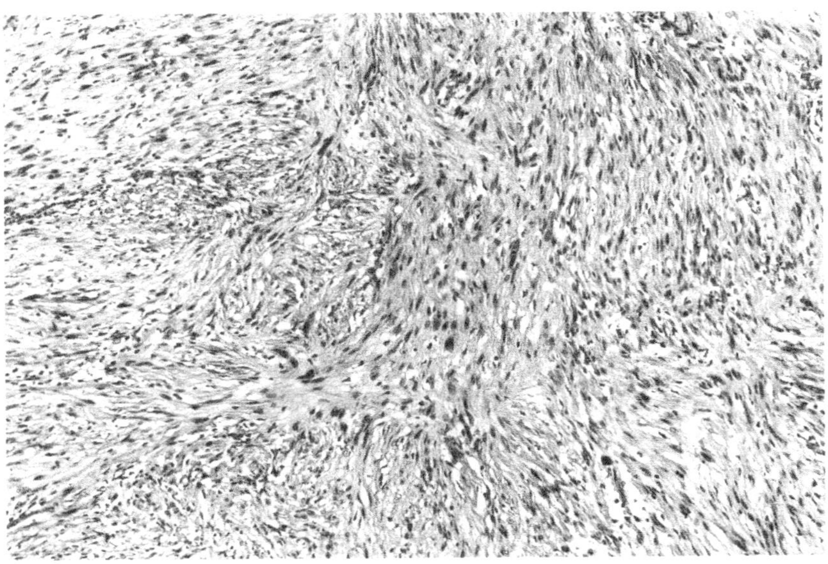

Fig. 86. *Neurilemmoma, stomach.* Compact spindle-cell area (Antoni A)

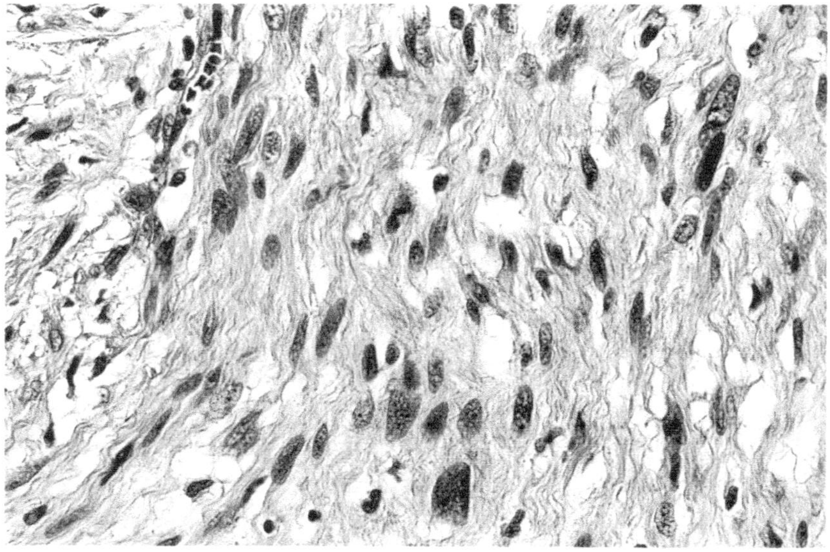

× 300

Fig. 87. *Neurilemmoma, stomach.* Wavy spindle cells with various sizes of nuclei and faintly eosinophilic cytoplasm. Same case as Fig. 86

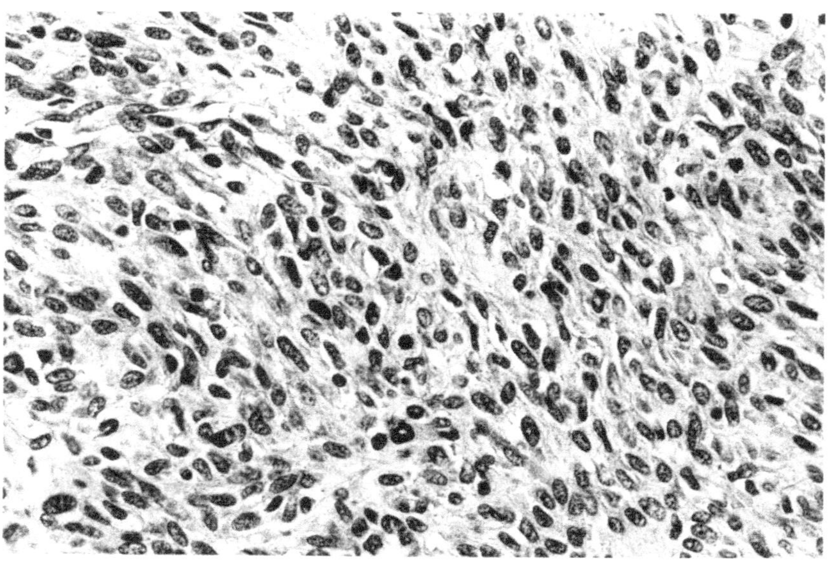

× 300

Fig. 88. *Leiomyosarcoma, stomach.* Mitoses

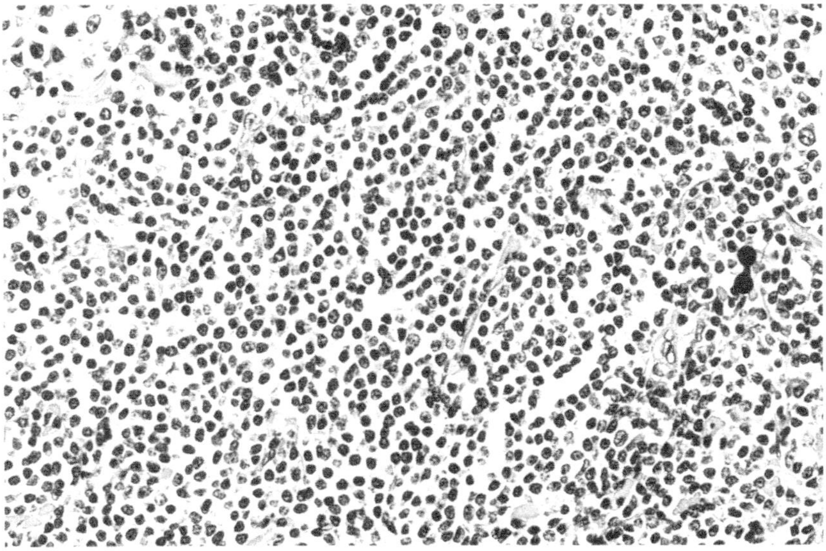

× 300

Fig. 89. *Malignant lymphoma, stomach.* Small lymphocytic

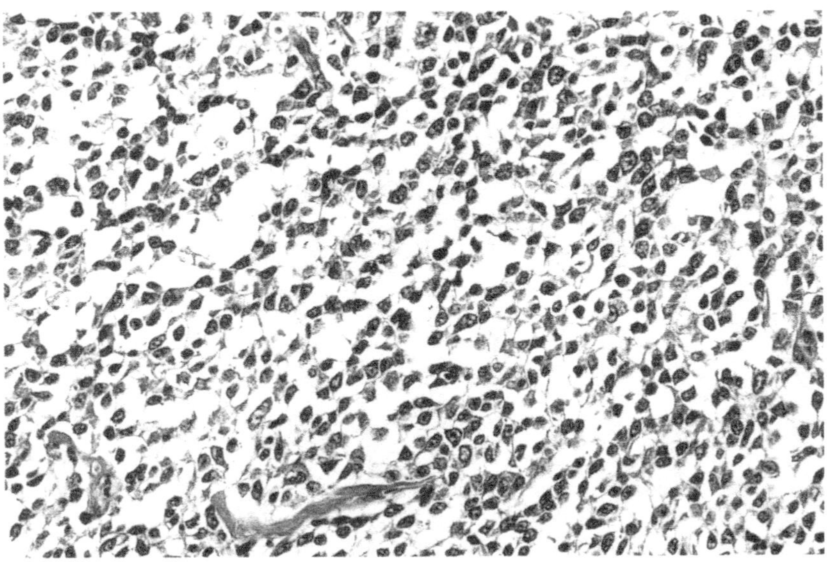

× 300

Fig. 90. *Malignant lymphoma, stomach.* Diffuse small cleaved cell

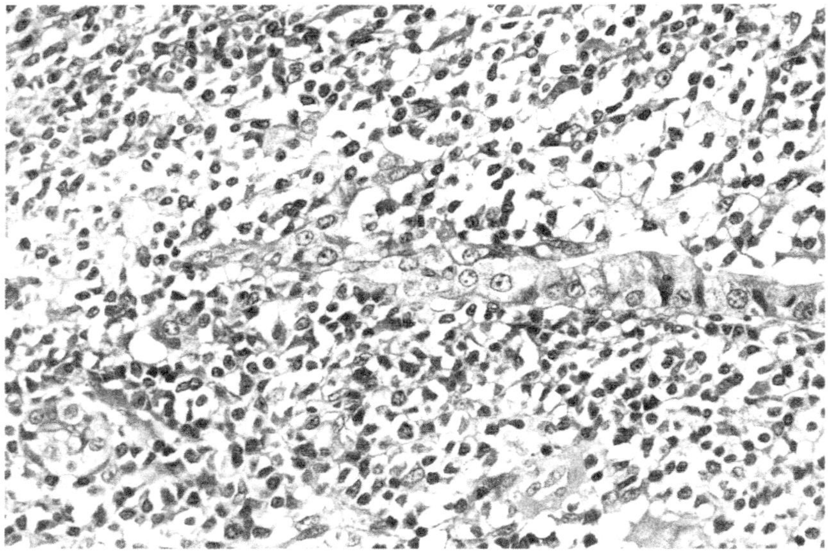

× 300

Fig. 91. *Malignant lymphoma, stomach.* Glands infiltrated and destroyed by lymphoid cells (lymphoepithelial lesion). Same case as Fig. 90

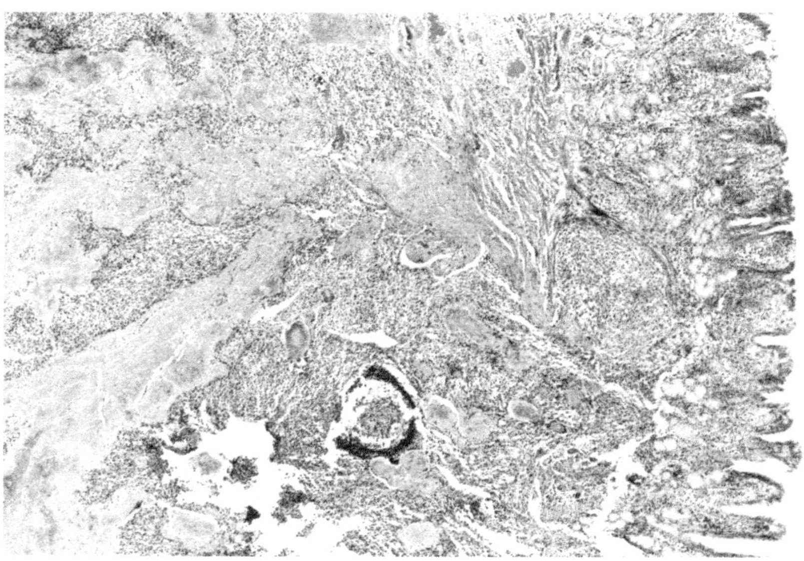

× 30

Fig. 92. *Plasmacytoma, stomach.* Associated amyloid deposits

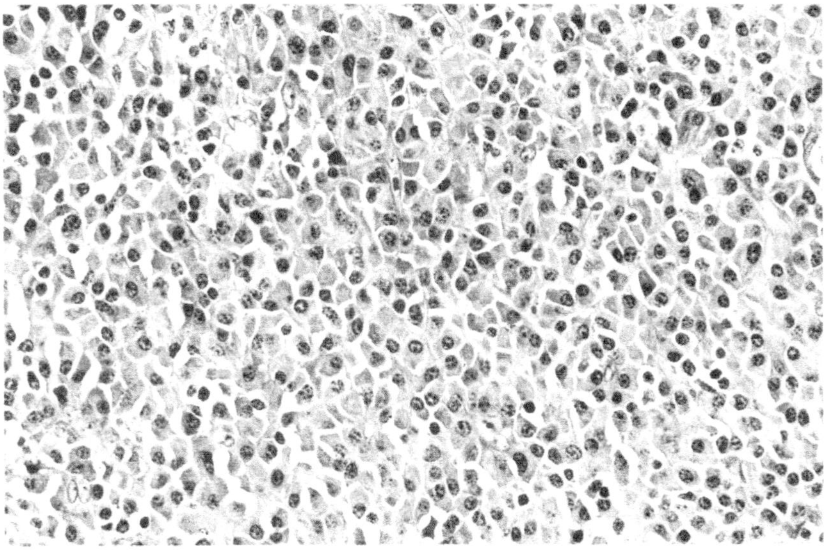

×300

Fig. 93. *Plasmacytoma, stomach.* Same case as Fig. 92

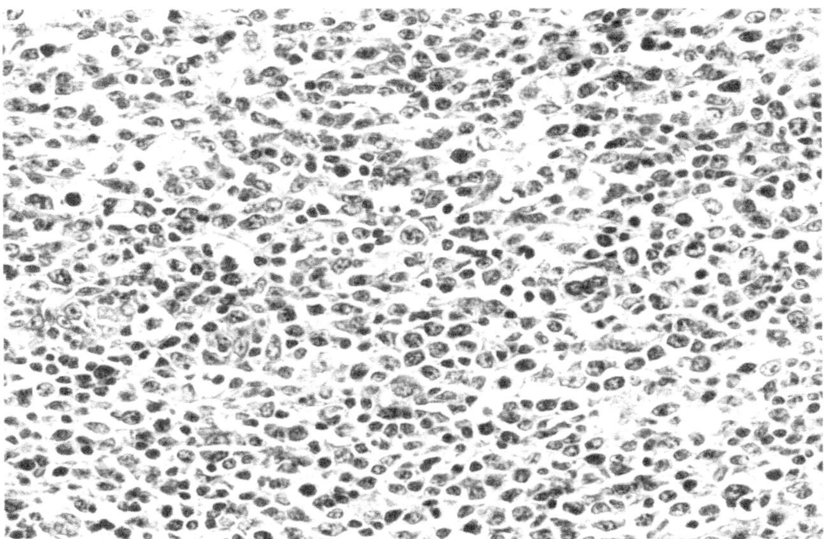

×300

Fig. 94. *Malignant lymphoma, stomach.* Follicular mixed small cleaved and large cell

×300

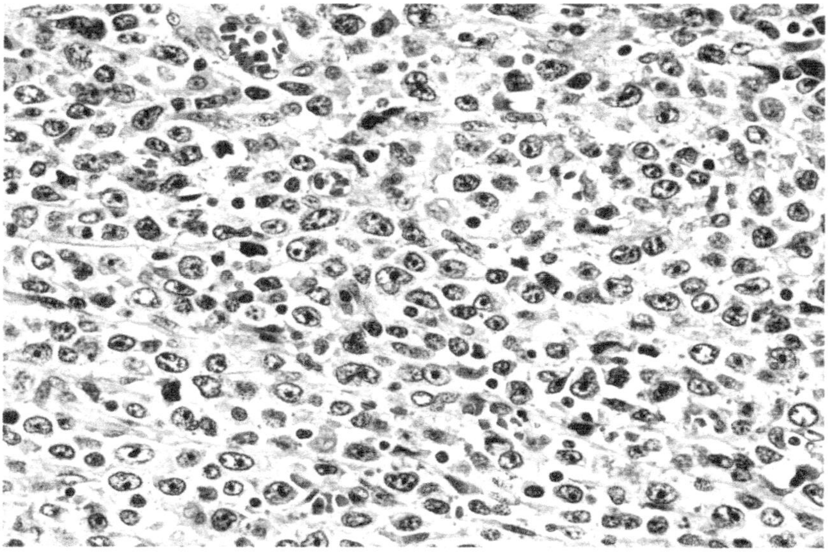

Fig. 95. *Malignant lymphoma, stomach.* Diffuse, large cell

×30

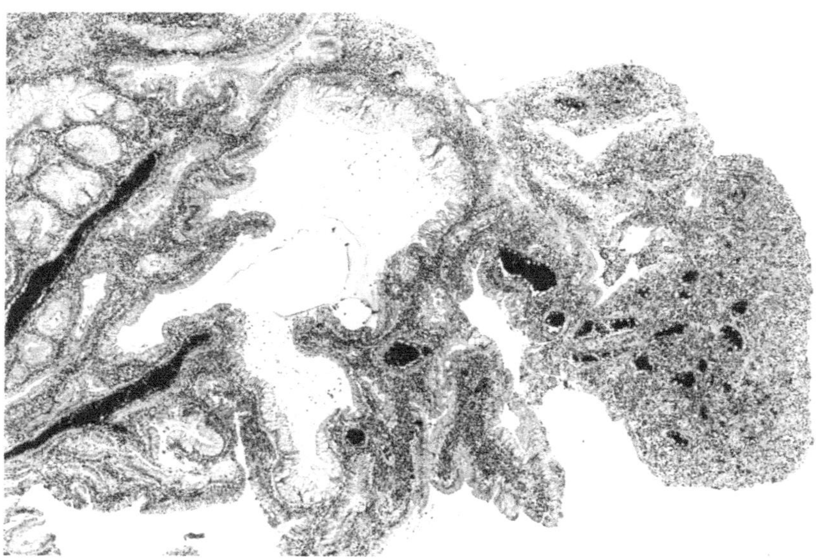

Fig. 96. *Hyperplastic polyp, stomach*

× 30

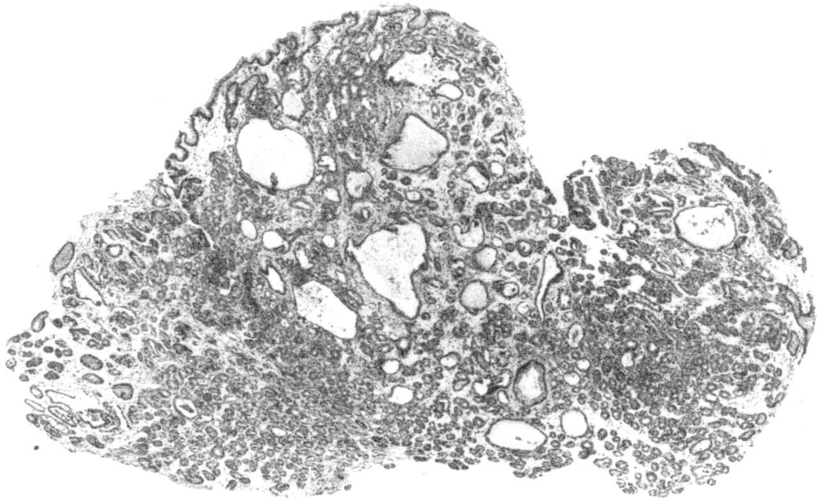

Fig. 97. *Fundic gland polyp, stomach.* Biopsy specimen from a 42-year-old woman without familial adenomatosis coli

× 150

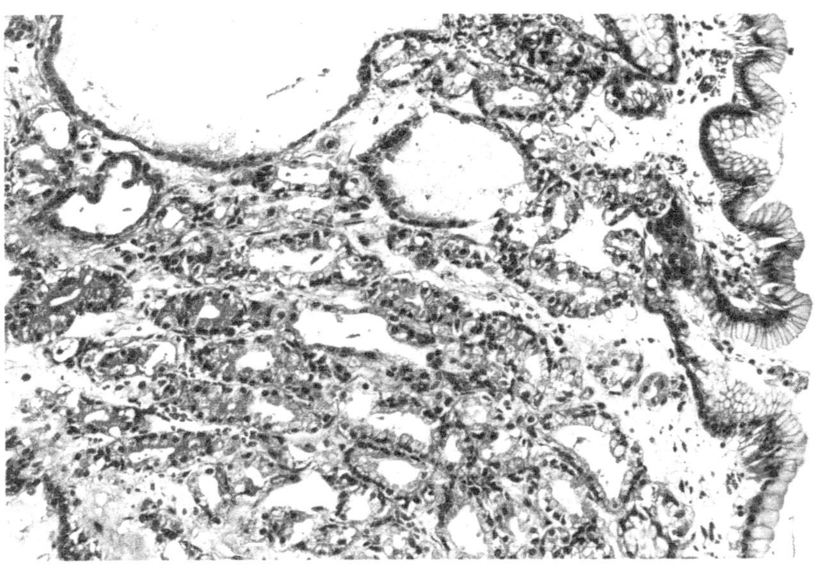

Fig. 98. *Fundic gland polyp, stomach.* Same case as Fig. 97

×8

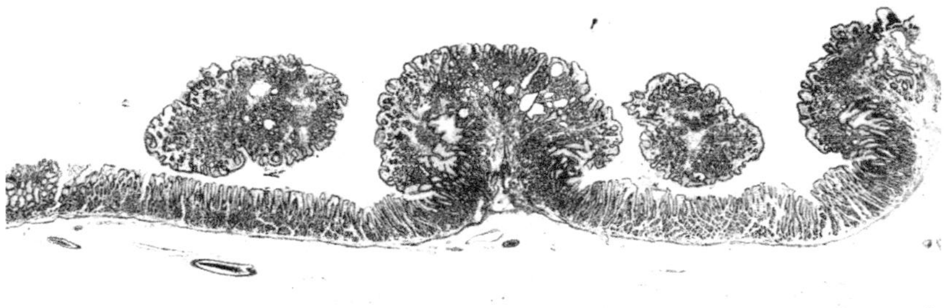

Fig. 99. *Fundic gland polyposis, stomach.* About 1880 polyps limited to gastric fundic mucosa of patient with familial adenomatosis coli

×30

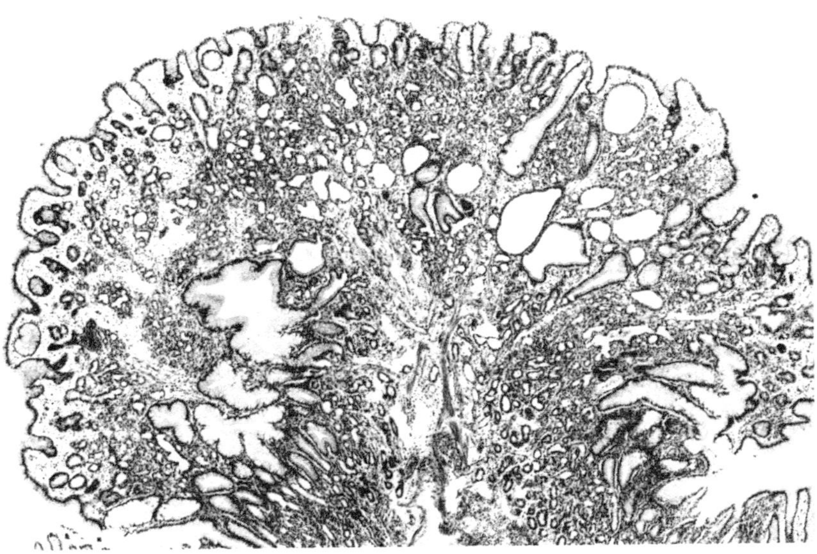

Fig. 100. *Fundic gland polyposis, stomach.* Same case as Fig. 99 (Colour illustration see p. 107)

×30

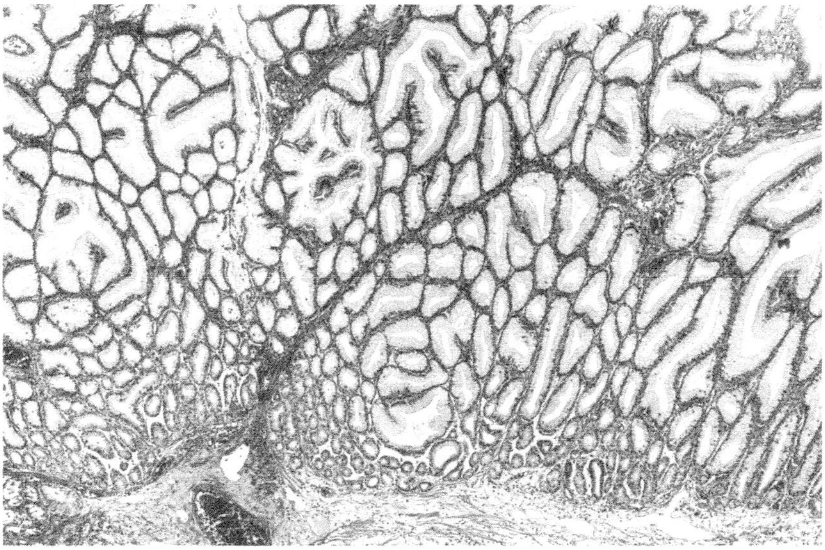

Fig. 101. *Peutz-Jeghers polyp, stomach.* Antral polyp with branching cores of muscularis mucosae and hyperplastic foveolae

×30

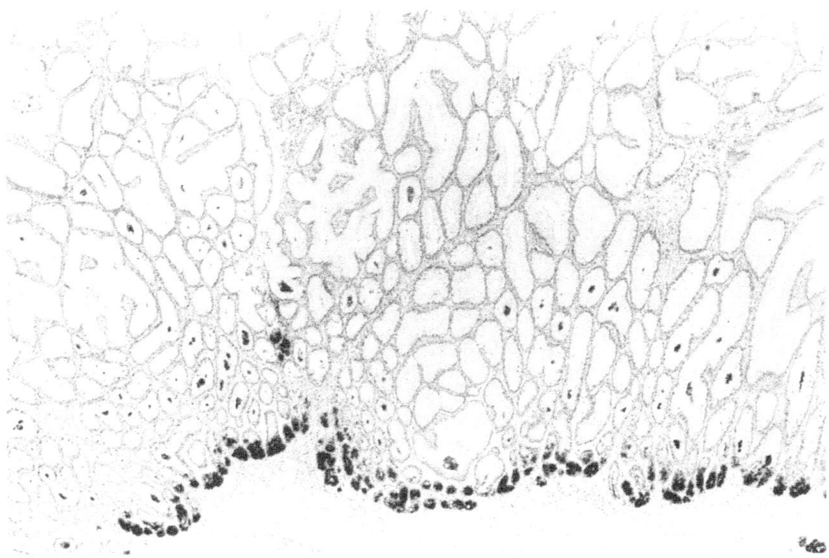

Fig. 102. *Peutz-Jeghers polyp, stomach.* Paradoxical concanavalin A staining positive for pyloric glands. Same case as Fig. 101

×8

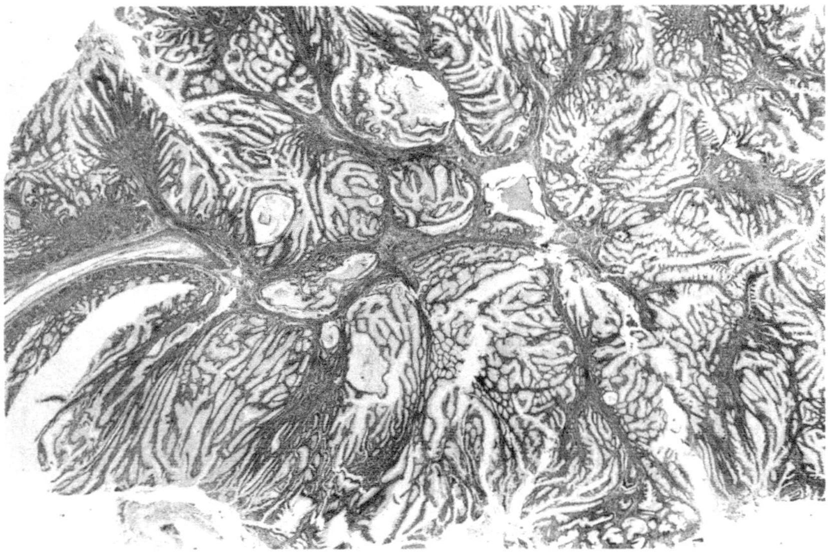

Fig. 103. *Peutz-Jeghers polyp, stomach.* Polyp arising from fundic mucosa. Branching core of muscularis mucosae with prominent foveolar hyperplasia

×8

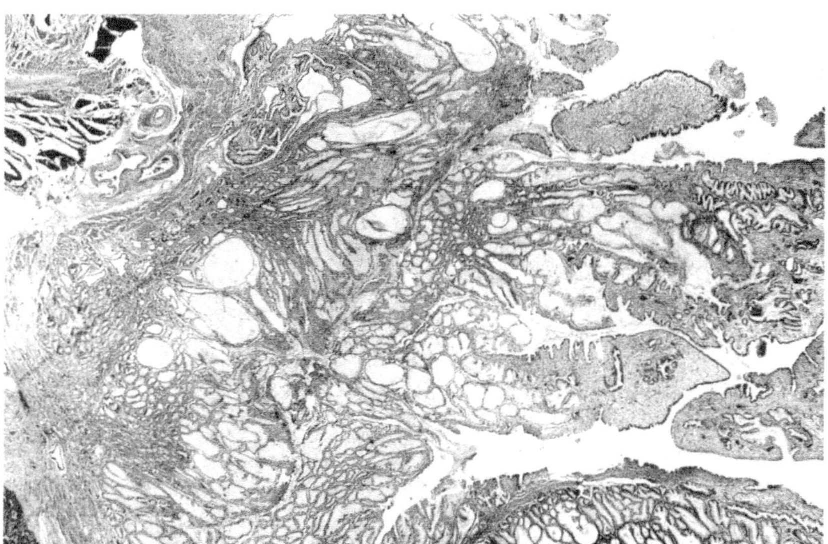

Fig. 104. *Juvenile polyposis, stomach.* Case of gastrointestinal juvenile polyposis

×75

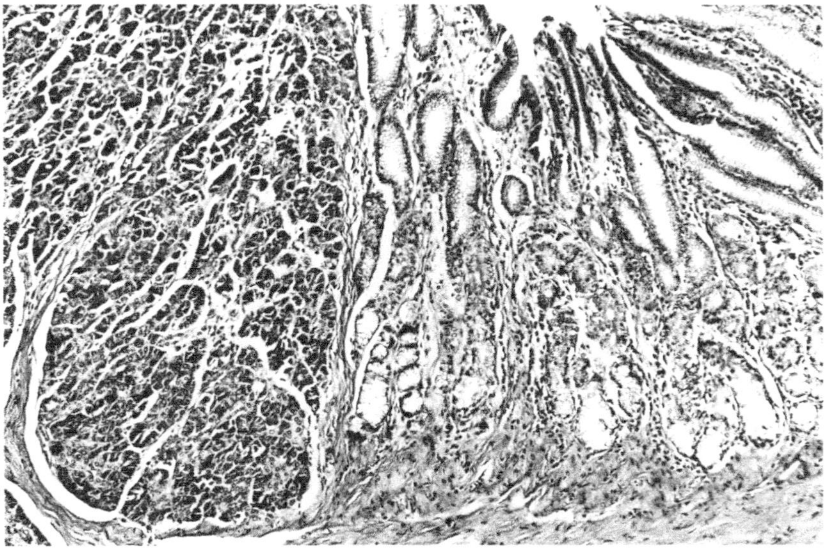

Fig. 105. *Pancreatic heterotopia, stomach.* Lesion located beneath mucosa as well

×30

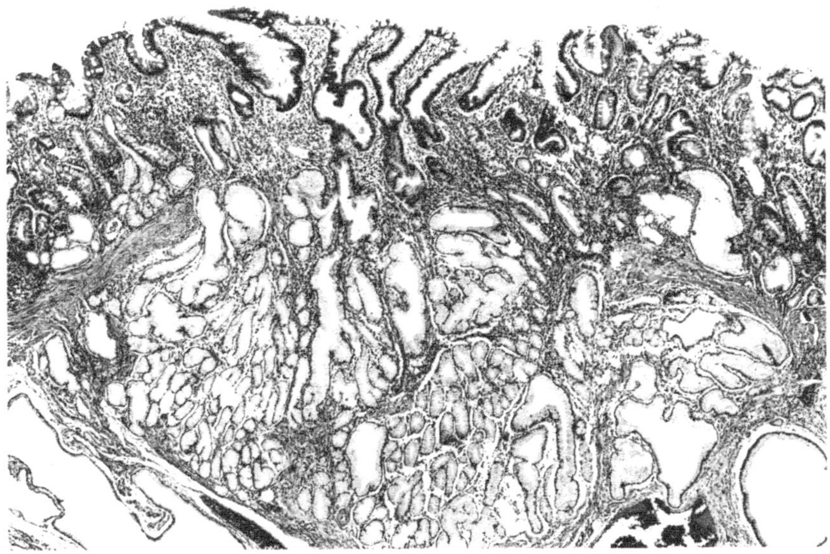

Fig. 106. *Gastric gland heterotopia, stomach*

×8

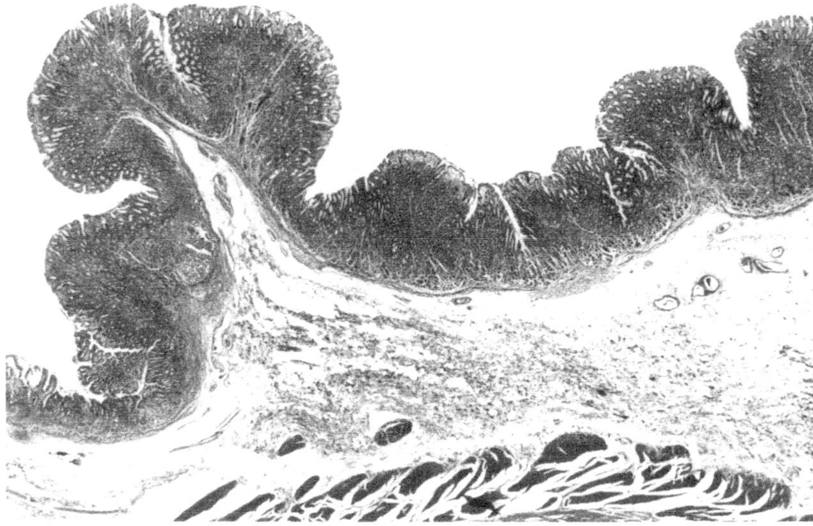

Fig. 107. *Giant rugal hypertrophy, stomach.* Balanced hyperplasia of fundic mucosa

×8

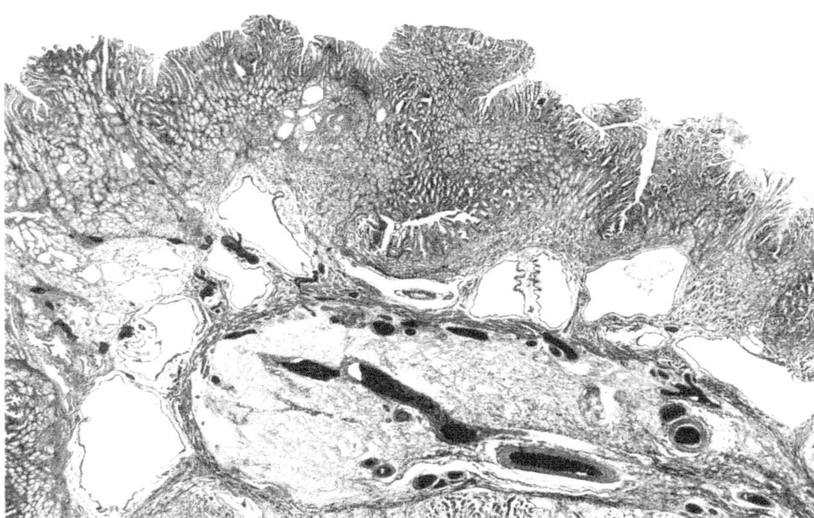

Fig. 108. *Giant rugal hypertrophy, stomach.* Pseudopyloric gland metaplasia and cystic change

×30

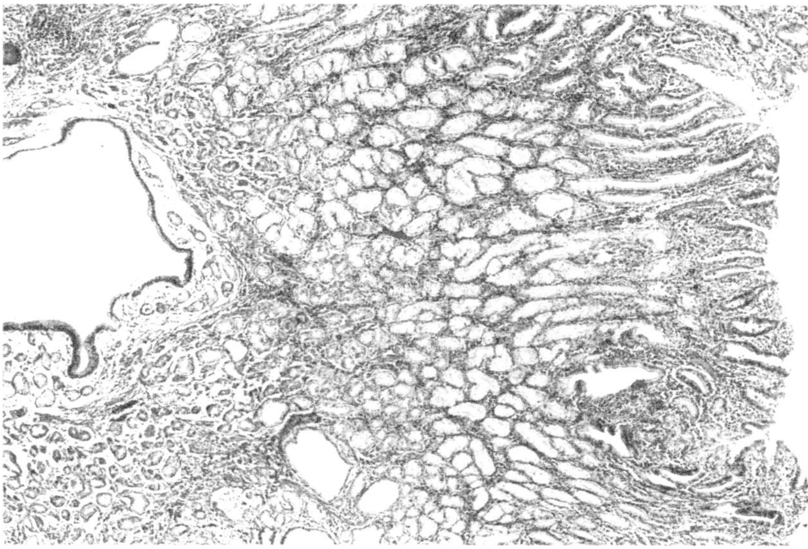

Fig. 109. *Giant rugal hypertrophy, stomach.* Same case as Fig. 108

×8

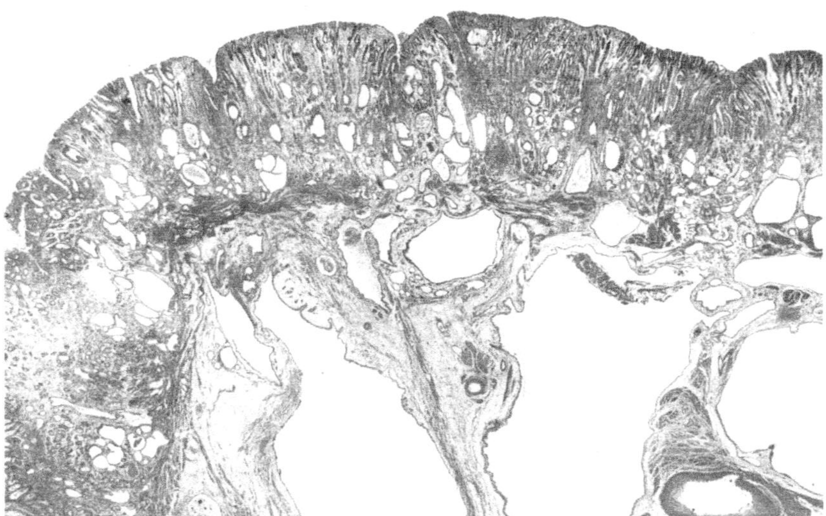

Fig. 110. *Gastritis cystica polyposa (stomal polypoid hypertrophic gastritis)*

×75

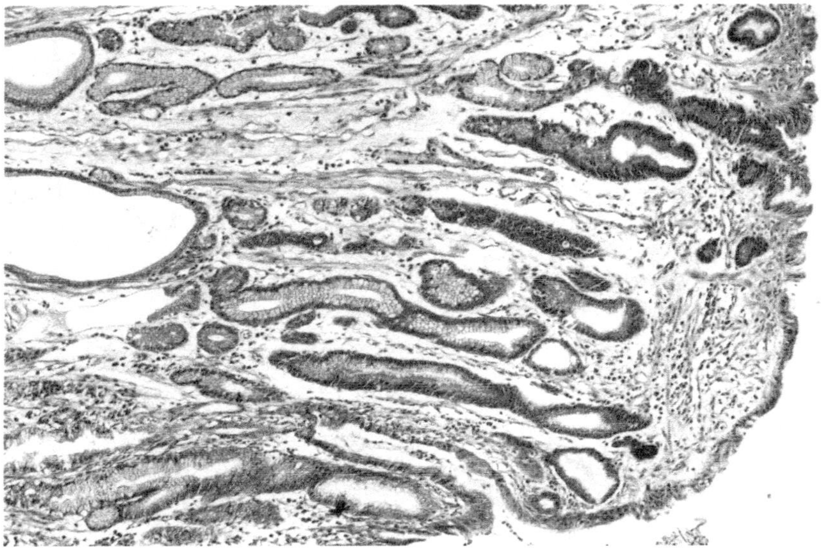

Fig. 111. *Gastritis cystica polyposa (stomal polypoid hypertrophic gastritis)* Same case as Fig. 110

×8

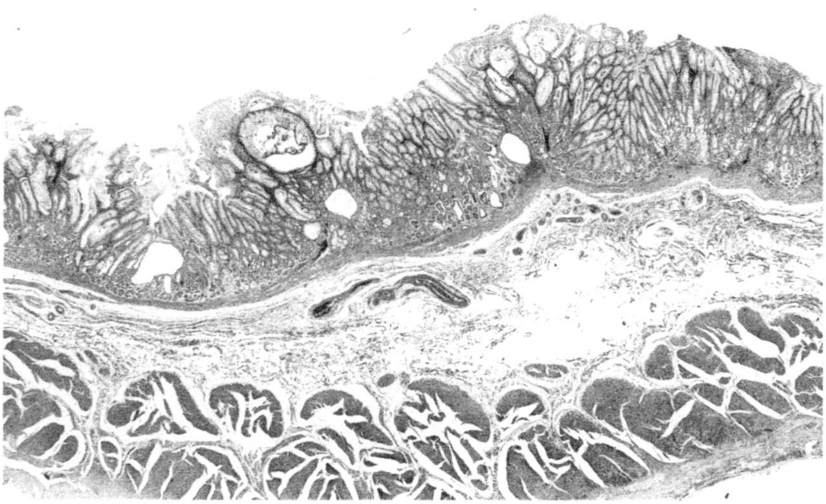

Fig. 112. *Cronkhite-Canada polyposis, stomach.* Autopsy of case treated medically

× 30

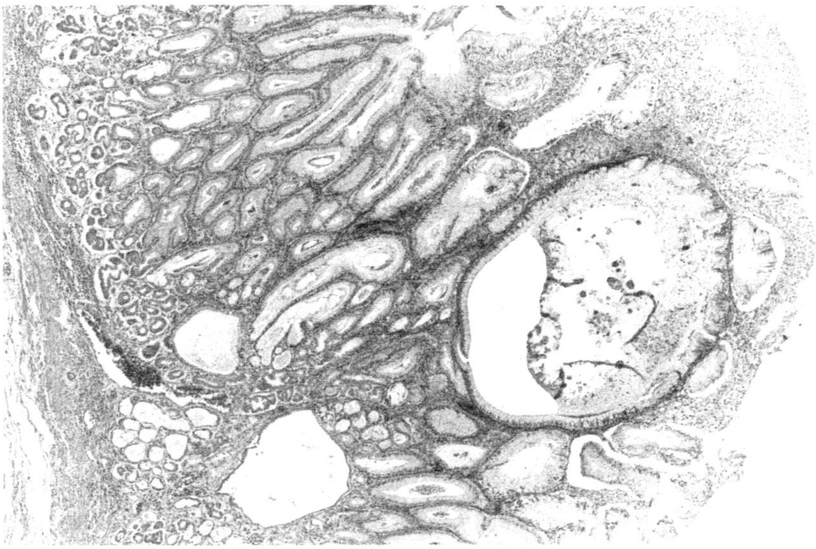

Fig. 113. *Cronkhite-Canada polyposis, stomach.* Same case as Fig. 112

× 30

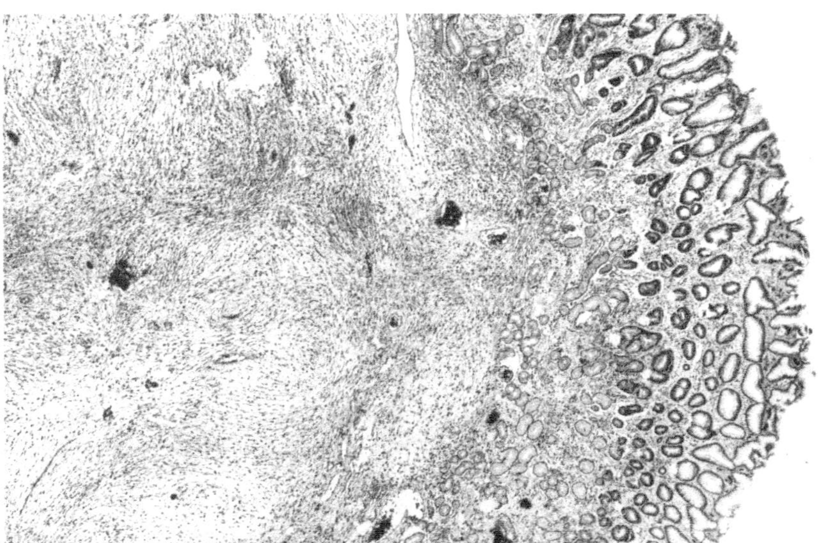

Fig. 114. *Inflammatory fibroid polyp, stomach*

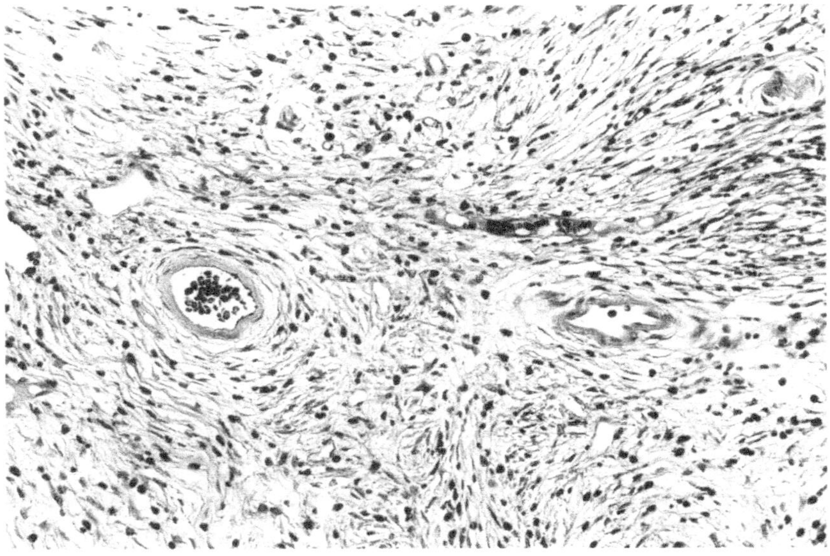

× 150

Fig. 115. *Inflammatory fibroid polyp, stomach.* Perivascular arrangement of fibroblasts (onion-skin pattern). Same case as Fig. 114
(Colour illustration see p. 107)

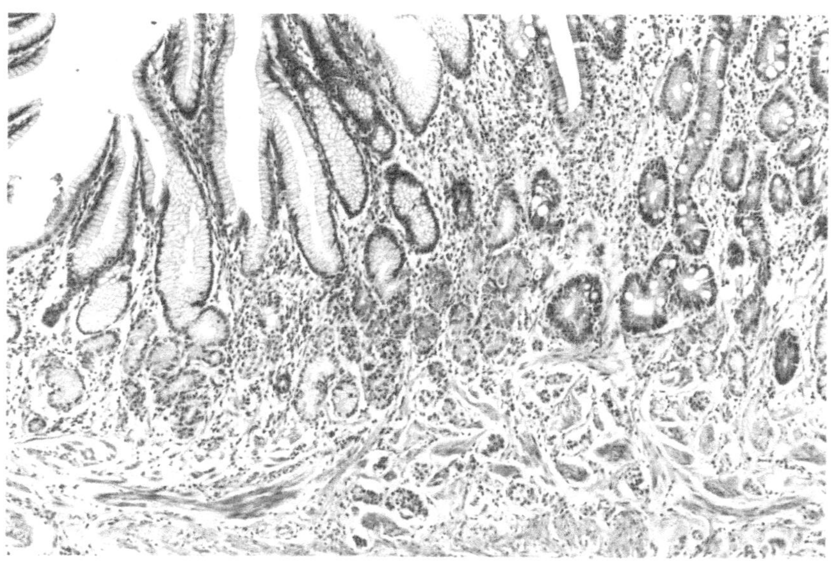

× 75

Fig. 116. *Endocrine cell hyperplasia and micronests, stomach.* Atrophic fundic mucosa of patient with pernicious anaemia (type A gastritis)
(Colour illustration see p. 108)

×75

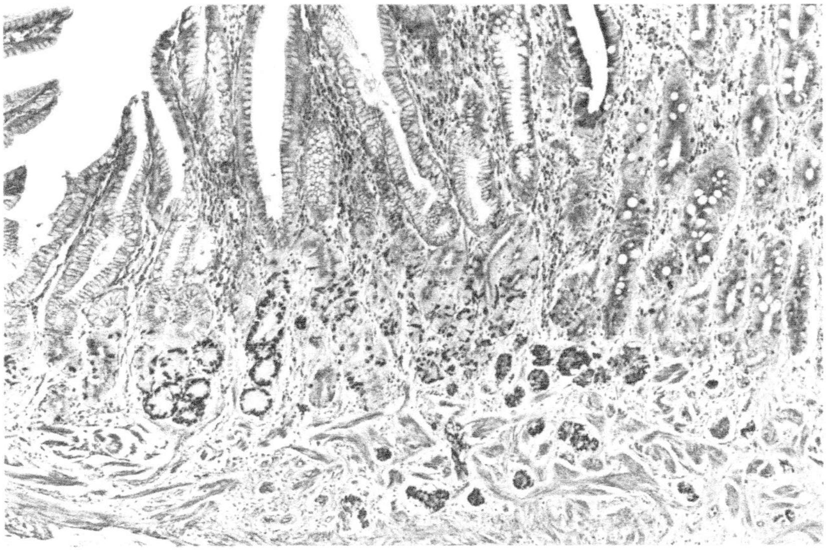

Fig. 117. *Endocrine cell hyperplasia and micronests, stomach.* Grimelius staining is positive *(black).* Endocrine cell hyperplasia in atrophic fundic glands and endocrine cell micronests in deep mucosa. Same case as Fig. 116
(Colour illustration see p. 108)

×8

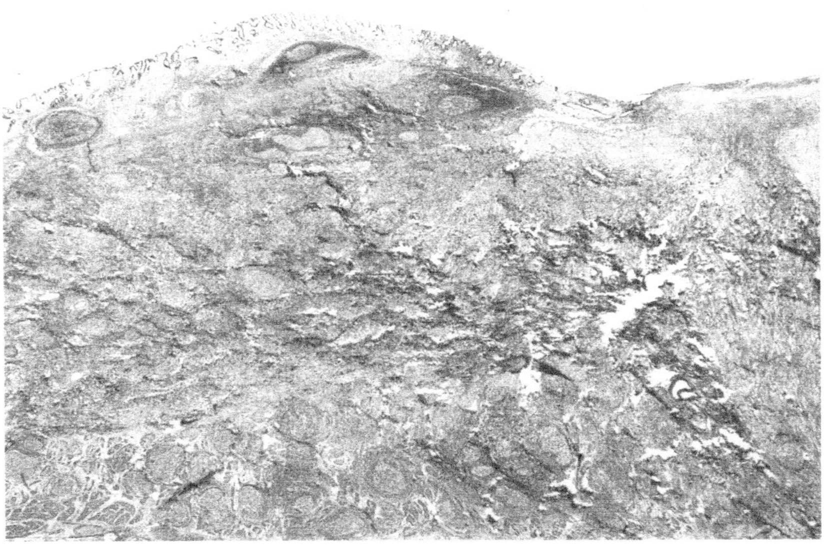

Fig. 118. *Benign lymphoid hyperplasia, stomach.* Ulceration at upper right

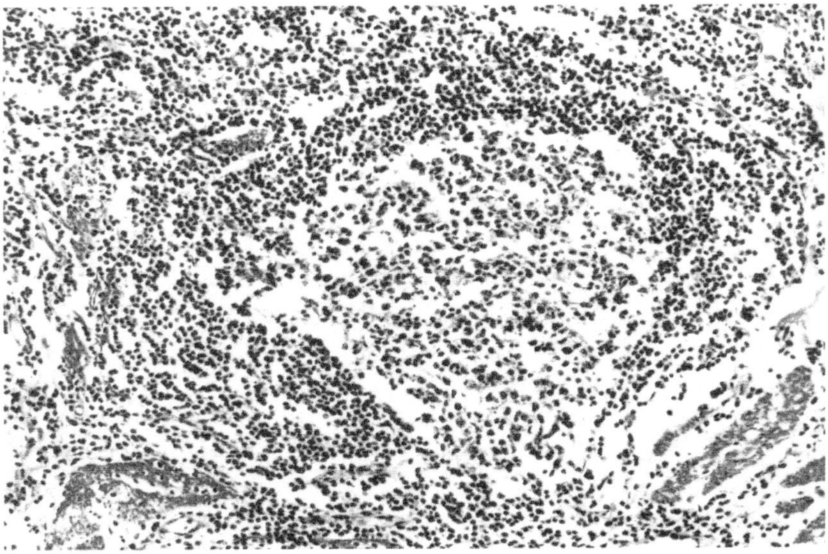

× 150

Fig. 119. *Benign lymphoid hyperplasia, stomach.* Well-outlined lymph follicle with distinct germinal centre. Same case as Fig. 118

× 8

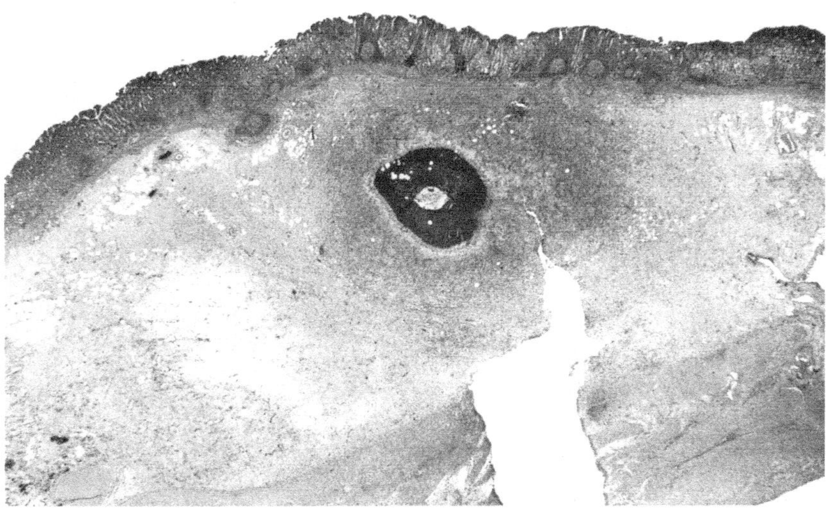

Fig. 120. *Anisakiasis, stomach.* Granulomatous stage

× 150

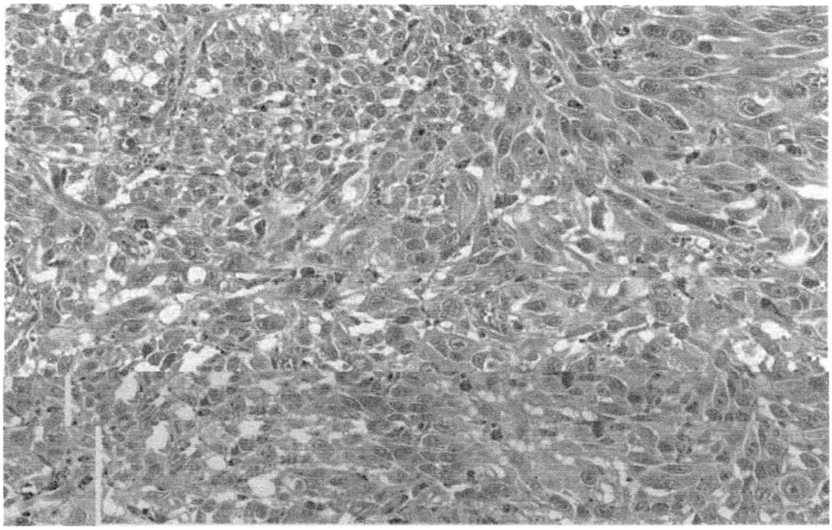

Fig. 23. *Malignant melanoma, oesophagus.* Melanin is seen

× 30

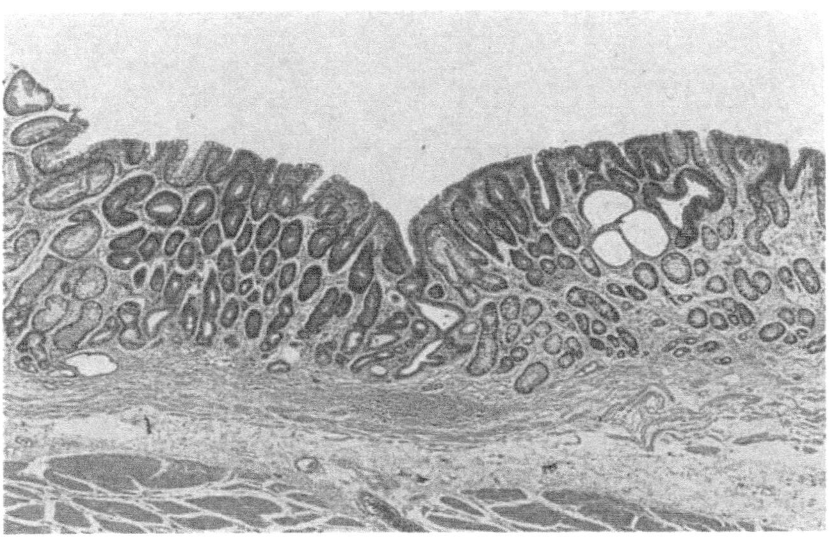

Fig. 35. *Tubular adenoma, stomach.* Depressed lesion measuring 2.7 × 2 mm

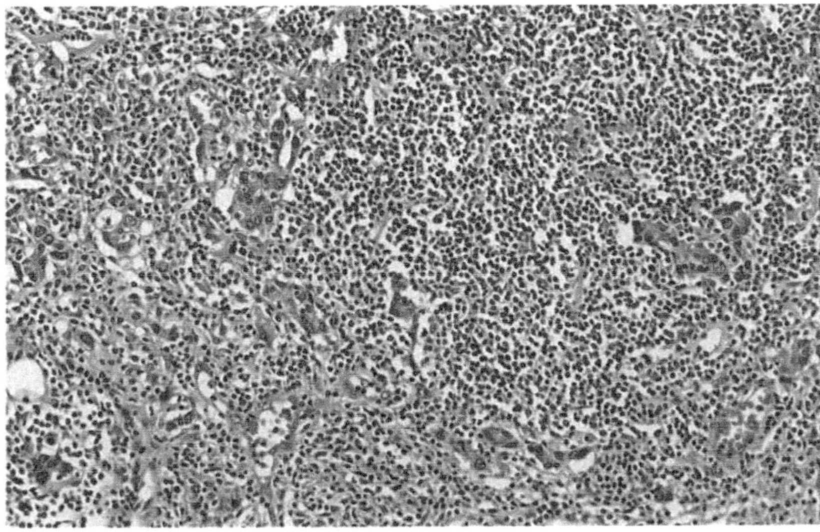

× 150

Fig. 61. *Tubular adenocarcinoma, stomach.* Poorly differentiated. Lymphoid stroma

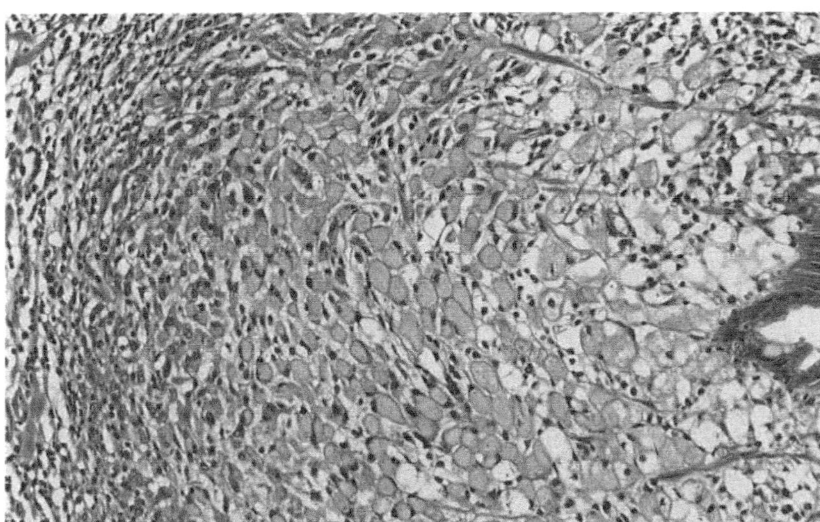

× 150

Fig. 64. *Signet-ring cell carcinoma, stomach.* Two-layered pattern in intramucosal carcinoma, 12 × 9 mm

× 30

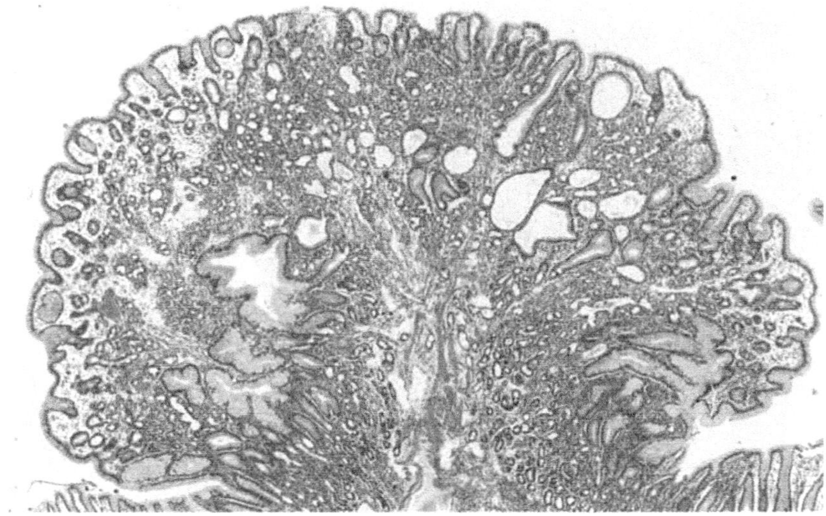

Fig. 100. *Fundic gland polyposis, stomach.* Same case as Fig. 99

× 150

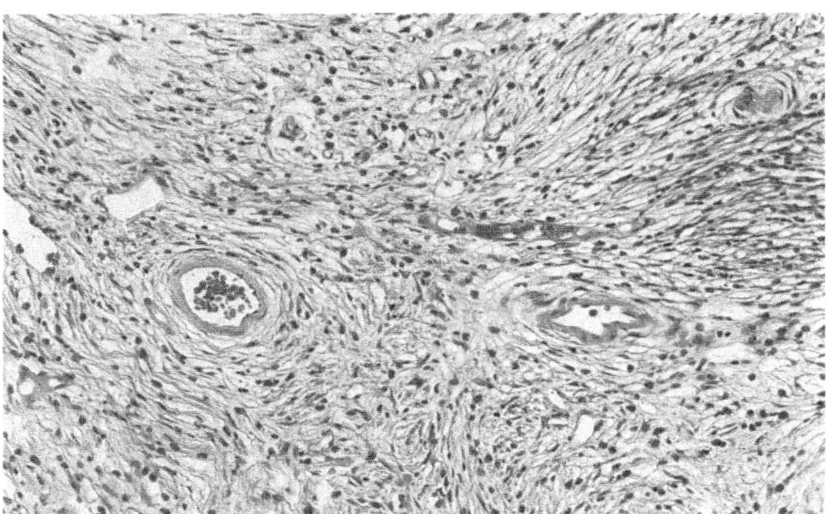

Fig. 115. *Inflammatory fibroid polyp, stomach.* Perivascular arrangement of fibroblasts (onion-skin pattern). Same case as Fig. 114

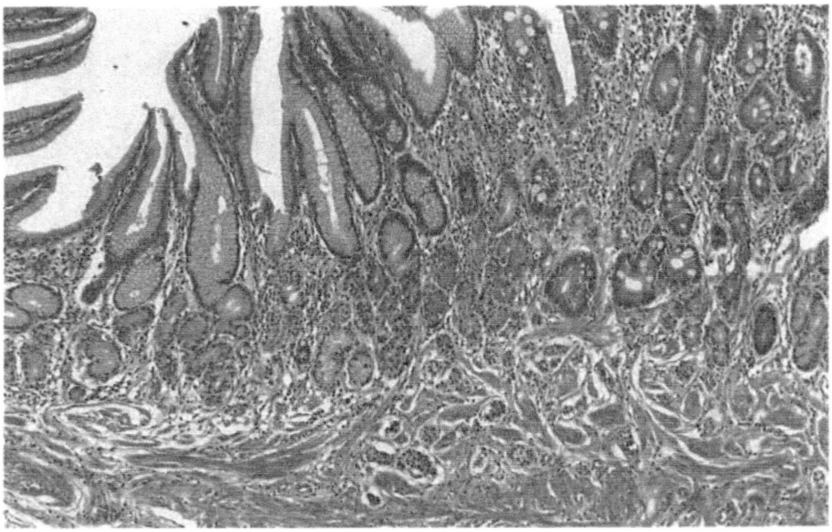

× 75

Fig. 116. *Endocrine cell hyperplasia and micronests, stomach.* Atrophic fundic mucosa of patient with pernicious anaemia (type A gastritis)

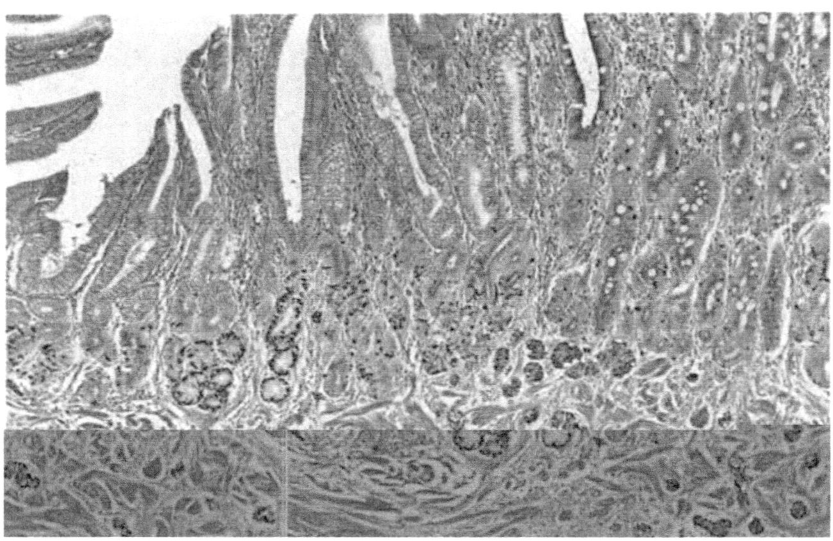

× 75

Fig. 117. *Endocrine cell hyperplasia and micronests, stomach.* Grimelius staining is positive *(black).* Endocrine cell hyperplasia in atrophic fundic glands and endocrine cell micronests in deep mucosa. Same case as Fig. 116

WHO International Histological Classification of Tumours
Watanabe, Jass and Sobin: Histological Typing of Oesophageal and Gastric Tumours, 2nd edn.

35 mm Color Transparencies

A set of 120 color slides (35 mm), corresponding to the photomicrographs in this book, is available from the American Registry of Pathology. To order these *slides,* send the following information to:

American Registry of Pathology
14th Street and Alaska Ave. NW
Washington, DC 20306 USA

Please send me:

_______ set(s) of 35 mm slides of Histological Typing of Oesophogeal and Gastric Tumors at $ 65.00 per set.
For Air Mail outside of North America add $ 10.00.

Total cost: $ _______ .00

Name ____

Address ____

____

____

Date ____________________ Signature ____________________

☐ I enclose a check/money order in US $ payable to the ARP.
☐ Please charge my credit card:
  ☐ VISA
    ☐ MasterCard

Card number ____

Expiration date ______________________________________

Name as it appears on credit card ______________________

Prices are subject to change without notice.

Batch number: 10723986

Printed by Printforce, the Netherlands